**By Christopher Dow**

*Fiction*
The Books of Bob
 Devil of a Time
 Jumping Jehovah
The Clay Guthrie Mysteries
 The Dead Detective
 Landscape with Beast
Roadkill
The Werewolf and Tide, and other Compulsions

*Nonfiction*
Lord of the Loincloth (nonfiction novel)
The Wellspring: An Inquiry into the Nature of Chi
Circling the Square: Observations on the Dynamics of Tai Chi Chuan
Elements of Power: Essays on the Art and Practice of Tai Chi Chuan
Alchemy of Breath: An Introduction to Chi Kung
Book of Curiosities: Adventures in the Paranormal

*Poetry*
City of Dreams
The Trip Out
Texas White Line Fever
Networks
Puzzle Pieces: Selected Poems

*Editor*
The Abby Stone: The Poetry of Bartholo Dias
The Best of Phosphene
The Best of Dialog

# Circling the Square

# Circling the Square

Observations on the Dynamics of Tai Chi Chuan

Christopher Dow

Phosphene Publishing Company
Houston, Texas

*Circling the Square: Observations on the Dynamics of Tai Chi Chuan*

© 2015 by Christopher Dow
ISBN: 0985147741
ISBN 13: 978-0-9851477-4-7

Published by:
Phosphene Publishing Company
Houston, Texas, USA
phosphenepublishing.com

2.1

For Dave Walker

# Contents

# Circling the Square

# Preface

**In modern times,** we've seen many changes in Tai Chi, and no less so for its introduction in the West. For that, we are indebted to exponents who traveled to China to study with masters there or who undertook extensive training under Chinese masters who had re-located to Europe and the Americas. Many of these people exhibit profound understanding of Tai Chi's underlying principles and utility and have continued the art's time-honored traditions even while expanding those traditions with fresh lines of inquiry and perceptive interpretations.

I was fortunate to have learned Tai Chi from three competent teachers who practiced solid, genuine forms and who wanted to share what they knew. I began studying Tai Chi in 1979 by learning Wu Family style from Frieda Armstrong Fox and other students of Li Li Da, a student of Wu Kung-i who taught in the San Francisco Bay area. Six years later, I began to study Northern Wu style with Dr. John Song, an acupuncturist and traditional Chinese physician, who learned from Lai De-ling, who learned from Wang Jun-sheng. This form, slightly modified, is the one I still practice. Dr. Song also taught me an excellent chi kung form, Xiao Style, which he learned from Xiao Liang-an and which I detail in my book, *Alchemy of Breath: An Introduction to Chi Kung*. A couple of years after that, I learned a fairly standard long version of Yang style from my friend Jack McGann, who studied, in part, with Benjamin Lo, one of Cheng Man-ching's foremost students.

I was unfortunate in that none of my teachers was then a master level expert, so their knowledge, while good to a point, was not deep enough at the time to allow them to explain or demonstrate Tai Chi's more profound functionality and energy work. To make matters worse, for much of the subsequent time I've practiced Tai Chi, I've done so in relative isolation. During those years, though, I managed to take workshops from some truly expert Tai Chi exponents, both Chinese and American. While I can't claim that any of the expertise of those sifus and masters actually rubbed off on me, the encounters did give me clues and insights into the art I've come to rely on as a cornerstone of my life. As have my readings on the subject and my observations of Tai Chi practitioners from many styles, both novice and expert. In this sense, the online video world—*YouTube*, etc.—is a godsend for Tai Chi practitioners because it facilitates the widespread dissemination of videos of what can only be called a dynamic art ill-served by static images. (Plenty of which the reader will find in this book!)

So, while I am certainly no master, I have spent considerable time practicing and studying the version of Tai Chi that I do, and my quest to understand more of this wonderful and profound art has led me to try to comprehend the principles I've read about and seen in other, more adept exponents and to integrate them into my own practice. In a sense, the lack of a truly expert, long-term teacher has worked to my advantage, for it forced me to seek the answers on my own instead of just learning rote lessons, and over the years, I have put a lot of work and thought into the matter of Tai Chi.

In another sense, my quest also became a validation of Tai Chi. If the art is true and real, it should, through time spent practicing its movements and contemplating its principles, teach even the most isolated sincere practitioner something that really works as an exercise, as a health maintenance system, and as a martial art. Through the years, Tai Chi has proved itself to me again and again. Indeed, over time, Tai Chi has become less of a something that I do and more of a something that always is within me.

As important as teachers, workshops, books, and videos have been to my Tai Chi development, just as significant were the several people I pushed hands extensively with with over the years. Nothing beats hands-on experience when dealing with a system of movement, particularly a martial art. I'm thinking of three of them in particular: Jack McGann, who taught me Yang style; Tony Ware, an Australian who learned Praying Mantis kung fu in his native country; and Dave Walker, who has a background in Tae Kwon Do, karate, and Northern Long Fist kung fu. I practiced form work, push hands, and applications for several years with each of them— and still do with Dave, though we're getting long in the tooth.

Occasionally when we've practiced, we've shown that the effort was worthwhile.

And as we gradually got a little better at what we were doing, I had the opportunity to work out some ideas that I was developing based on my observations of our form and push hands work and through observations of the forms and push hands abilities of Tai Chi players of superior stature than ours. My deepest thanks and regards to each of them and to everyone I've had the privilege to learn from, be they true masters of the art or my beginner students.

My book, *The Wellspring: An Inquiry into the Nature of Chi*, discussed the human body's energy—chi—and its methods of generation and mobilization. In the present volume, I want to examine Tai Chi dynamics, which range from several aspects of physical movement to the impact those movements can have at the more subtle energy level of chi.

To tell the truth, though, I'm writing this book as much to work out and organize my thoughts on Tai Chi as I am for any other purpose. It's probably a futile effort, though. Tai Chi is too deep and wide to encompass—at least with words and pictures. Words and pictures merely stand facing the great Tai Chi sea and imagine they see a distant shore where marvels glitter. But that distant shore might be no less a mirage than are distant lakes shimmering on a desert's horizon.

But I guess I can't help but try to comprehend as much as I can of Tai Chi, which seems to work whether you consciously understand it or not. It's so interesting to try to figure out. Even better, when I look around at others in my age group, I see that I'm in pretty good shape compared to most of them. I also can sometimes sense or notice what many of them can't. And I'm not knocking Tai Chi's self-defense aspect or leaving it until last because it's least. It isn't. Instead, it is, I think, crucial to learning what Tai Chi is about because, even if fighting isn't the practitioner's purpose, the martial applications have specific goals and thus can inform one about what is—or should be—going on inside the body when executing a given movement, and it also can be used as a method to learn to lead the chi through the body. But fighting is, after all, such a small sliver of reality. For me, what's truly beneficial about Tai Chi, aside from its value as physical and energetic exercise, is that it encourages me to investigate the nature of reality and to open myself to its manifold wonders.

I credit Tai Chi for the many aids it has given my life, and because Tai Chi works in several very different but interlinked ways, my mind wants to know how and why it works. Hence this book, which is simply a proposal regarding conclusions that I've come to by using my own body as a laboratory. I'm not saying that my conclusions are the lodestar that invariably points to the "real" way Tai Chi works. I don't know what real Tai Chi is for others. I only know what Tai Chi is to me. So this book describes the way I think Tai Chi works. But like I said, that distant shore might be a mirage....

Six in the second place means:
Straight, square, great.
Without purpose,
Yet nothing remains unfurthered.

The symbol of heaven is the circle, and that of earth is the square. Thus square-ness is a primary quality of the earth. On the other hand, movement in a straight line, as well as magnitude, is a primary quality of the Creative. But all square things have their origin in a straight line and in turn form solid bodies.

—I Ching[1]

# Notes on Methodology

**Before we begin,** I want to explain a few technical matters that pertain to this book. The first is terminology. For the most part, I will use the English terms for the Thirteen Postures rather than the Chinese. I have a couple of reasons for doing this. First, I am writing in English for an English-reading audience. Second, the concepts are difficult enough without having to memorize words in a language one does not understand, and my purpose here is to explicate rather than obscure.

Some people will argue that the English terms do not fully represent the concepts found in the Chinese terms. There is, in almost every translation of the Tai Chi Classics, a statement to this effect from the translator. This may be technically true, but my counterargument is that the intricacies of the word "Peng," and its ideogram for example, are lost on the English speaker, anyway. Ward Off serves just as well as Peng as a designator for the English speaker since the basic dynamics of Peng are not linguistic but mental and physical. If you understand within your mind and body what Peng is, then it doesn't really matter what you call it. Besides, Peng is a made-up word in Chinese, anyway, coined within the martial arts community specifically to describe the power produced by Tai Chi. Or, to use another example, it is definitely more descriptive for an English speaker to use the term Roll Back instead of Lu.

But I'd be foolish to insist on sticking to that formula when it won't work or isn't more illustrative than an existing Chinese word. There are plenty of Chinese martial arts terms for which there are no English equivalents. So far, no one has come up with a common English substitute for "fa jin"—the term used to indicate the manifestation of Tai Chi power—so in that case, I will use the Chinese term.

The idea of fa jin brings also up the use of the word Peng in a different context than its use to name the specific movement of Ward Off. The word Peng also is used to designate the condensed energy that supports fa jin. In this sense, Peng is in every Tai Chi movement, not just in Ward Off, and I'd like to reserve the word to identify that underlying energy rather than to indicate a specific movement.

I'll also use the word "tantien," which is used to name three power centers in the body: the brain, the heart, and most specifically, an area located approximately two inches below the navel and about one third of the distance behind the front of the torso toward the back. There is no English word for this third tantien because Western science does not acknowledge its existence. Since I covered the tantien's physiological existence and operation in *The Wellspring*, I won't go into it here but will assume that any reader familiar with Tai Chi also is familiar with the concept of the tantien.

Also, as you might already have noticed, I'm going to capitalize a lot of names that aren't always capitalized, such as the names of various martial arts styles. Tai Chi is one of those, but when I'm referring to the tai chi symbol, I'm going to lower case the term, since it is used in that instance to designate a philosophical concept rather than as a proper name for a particular martial art style. I'll also capitalize the names of the Cardinal and Ordinal Energies and the Five Steps because these refer to specific elements and concepts as distinguished from more general ones: You use Push to push.

As a final note on nomenclature, I want to point out one benefit to translating a Chinese term into English: You can get something quite poetic. Chinese speakers can only call the art Tai Chi Chuan. English speakers can call it Tai Chi Chuan, too, and most do, but we have some other very cool choices: Grand Ultimate Fist, Celestial Boxing, and one of my personal favorites, Primordial Pugilism.

The second matter is the many descriptions of Tai Chi movements in the pages that follow. To help explain concepts, I've tried to choose movements that both illustrate the concepts and are common to most Tai Chi styles, and I've used some of them to illustrate multiple concepts. While I might have made the right choices in most cases, it is entirely possible that other examples might better illustrate what I'm talking about. I apologize in advance for my failings. In addition, I've explained the movements well as I could, but truthfully, many Tai Chi movements are so complex that it is difficult to parse them in a strictly verbal manner. Worse, for me, is the fact that many movements embody multiple elements that can make them examples of entirely opposing concepts. In such cases, I've simply ignored one or more in favor of the one I'm trying to illustrate. I hope that, in the end, my choices and efforts will at least explain what I'm talking about well enough that the reader can extrapolate to other aspects of a movement or to other movements in his or her own form.

In a related matter, this book contains many illustrations, some of which are static images of objects and figures, while others are sort of slow-motion figure animations of Tai Chi movements. Please don't think that the figure illustrations—either static or moving—depict perfection of Tai Chi form. I certainly don't! I am not an exemplar of Tai Chi excellence. But I think they are suggestive enough to show what I'm talking about, so please forgive my postural lapses.

And finally, there are a number of references to the Tai Chi Classics. I've put them all into quotes to clarify that they are statements from the Classics, but that doesn't mean that all of them are direct quotes from specific translations. In some cases they are, and those are accompanied by footnotes. In other cases, I'm simply paraphrasing from memory general concepts elucidated by the Classics. I encourage the reader to absorb as much as possible from these seminal works on Tai Chi and to read as many translations of them as one can. Each is different and can bring fresh insights into the art of Tai Chi, especially those accompanied by commentary from an expert. I have my favorites, I read them frequently, and I'm sometimes pleased to discover that some statement in them that once was obscure now makes sense.

Squaring the Circle: The ancient Mesopotamians used to place a circle between two squares in order to find out its area. And the idea of equating the circle with the square also grew out of the concept of the rotating square. But our concern is not with the mathematical but the symbolic problem. 'Squaring the circle', like the *lapis* or the *aurum philosophicum*, was one of the preoccupations of the alchemists; but whereas the latter two were symbols of the quest for the evolutive goal of the spirit, the former problem concerned the equating of the two great cosmic symbols of heaven (or the circle) and earth (or the square). It is to do, then, with the union of two opposites; not juxtaposition as in the *coniunctio* of the two arms of the cross, for example, but the equation and cancelling out of two components in a higher synthesis. The square was seen to correspond to the four Elements. The aim of 'squaring the circle', then (which strictly ought to be called 'circling the square'), was to obtain unity in the material world (as well as in the spiritual life) over and above the differences and obstacles (the static order) of the number four and the four-cornered square. We have already suggested that the rotated square was reckoned an important part of this project, and Heinrich Khunrath comments in his *Von hylealischen Chaos*: 'By means of circumrotation or circulatory revolution, the quarternary is restored to purest simplicity and innocence'. Another means of getting an ersatz 'squaring' was to superimpose two squares, inscribing a circle within them, in such a way as to form an octagon. The octagon can indeed be considered, in both a geometric and a symbolic sense, as the intermediary form between the square and the circle. For this reason it never symbolized the *opus* itself (that is, the mystic consummation of the synthesis of opposites), but it did stand for a path indicated by things quarternary (such as the earth, the feminine element, matter or reason) towards the circle (representing perfection, eternity and spirit). That is why many mediaeval baptisteries, fonts and cupolas are octagonal in shape.

—J. E. Cirlot[42]

# Introduction

The dome of heaven rests on the quarters of the earth, sometimes supported by four caryatidal kings, dwarfs, giants, elephants, or turtles. Hence, the traditional importance of the mathematical problem of the quadrature of the circle: it contains the secret of the transformation of heavenly into earthly forms.

—Joseph Campbell[2]

**Tai Chi Chuan** is many things: a martial art, a mode of meditation, and a method to build internal vitality, strength, and power and, by extension, improve health. Ideally, all of these aspects interlink within the practitioner. We know that Tai Chi emerged into public view in the Chen Village of Henan Province in China in the seventeenth century, although legend and Chinese "Wild History" take it back in time another five hundred years to a Taoist monk named Chang San-feng. Chang supposedly created Tai Chi after witnessing a fight between a snake and a bird and noting that the snake's sinuous movements not only easily deflected the bird's swift and powerful strikes, but also provided the snake with a means to counterattack and defeat the bird.

One version of the art's subsequent dissemination has it that Chang passed his art on to others until it finally reached Wang Tsung-yueh and his disciple, Chiang Fa. One or the other of these men—both of whom reputedly made their livings as itinerant martial artists

—was passing through Henan Province and, while in Chen Village, made disparaging remarks about the Chen family's native martial art. Promptly challenged to prove himself, Wang (or Chiang) defeated all who fought him, and for a time, he stayed at the Chens' request to teach them his art.

The Chens deny this story and claim that Chen Wang-ting (1580-1660) was the founder of the art now known as Tai Chi. Perhaps they are right. But the tale of Wang Tsung-yueh is lent some credibility by the fact that Chen historical records do not mention Tai Chi or any similar art before the seventeenth century. It is as if Tai Chi suddenly appeared full-blown in Chen Village in the person of Chen Wang-ting, without prior development. In addition, there exist in the area of Chen Village several martial arts that are extremely similar to Tai Chi and that

**Figure 1** The tai chi symbol depicts the major forces of opposition and cooperation that underlie the functioning of reality.

have equally long histories, such as the martial art of nearby Zhaobao Village. The existence of these and other clues gives some credence to the idea that someone—Wang, Chiang, or someone else—traveled through the area, disseminating an art that eventually became Tai Chi. For an excellent analysis of these and other historical issues, see Douglas Wile's *Lost T'ai-chi Classics from the Late Ch'ing Dynasty*.

History is like a root that grows smaller and more obscure the farther you trace it, finally disappearing into the depths of the mysterious and impenetrable past. We probably will never know who originated Tai Chi. This adds to the art's mystique, lending it a sense of emerging directly from the Tao as a gift to humankind. At the same time, we can acknowledge that almost all current Tai Chi forms derive from Chen style. It is the trunk that produced Tai Chi's four major branches—Yang, Hao, Wu, and Sun—and numerous subbranches in the forms of shortened and hybrid styles. This proliferation of styles, however, only serves to highlight the question: What exactly *is* Tai Chi?

Obviously, Tai Chi is not a particular form or a specific set of movements, otherwise there would be only one version instead of the variety we now see. But the efficacy of these many styles—several of which are very different in appearance, "flavor," and even specific points of utility—indicates that each has something that can be called "tai chi."

Prior to the turn of the nineteenth century, the art was called, among other

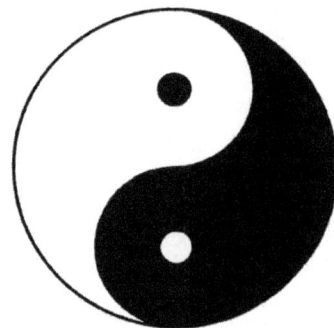

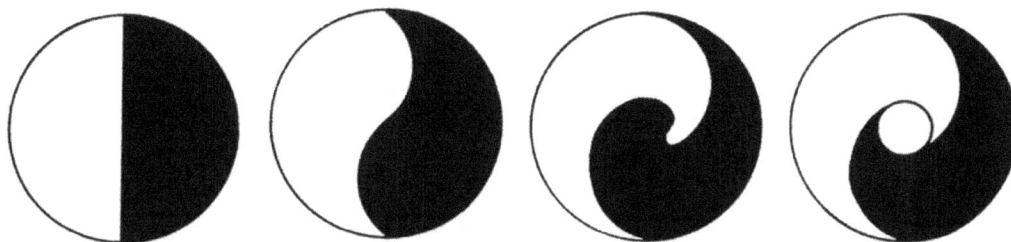

Figure 2 The tai chi symbol's wavy line demonstrates movement not just in space, but over time. The vortex that can develop in the center, like the eye of a hurricane, epitomizes the core of emptiness or tranquility the underlies all action.

names, Chen boxing, soft boxing (because of the relaxed execution of its solo form), long boxing (because of the relatively long solo practice routine), or often, the Thirteen Postures, which refers to the sum of Tai Chi's four Cardinal (principal) Energies, four Ordinal (ancillary) Energies, and Five Stances (the five basic directions of movement). These thirteen elements comprise the basic precepts by which Tai Chi operates, and all of them will be examined during the course of this book.

Then, as one story goes, in the mid 1800s, a scholar in the Imperial Court named Ong Tong He witnessed a demonstration match by the great and undefeated Tai Chi exponent and founder of Yang style, Yang Lu-chan. After the match, Ong wrote: "Hands holding Taiji shakes the whole world, a chest containing ultimate skill defeats a gathering of heroes."[3]

Ong could have been referring to the fluidity of Yang's movements or to the interplay of solidness and emptiness those movements demonstrated. But perhaps Ong saw beneath the surface to understand the way the art embodies the dynamics of movement and physical reality as expressed by the tai chi symbol. This symbol depicts in two dimensions—height and width—a sphere that epitomizes the major forces of opposition and cooperation that underlie the functioning of three-dimensional reality. (Figure 1) It also defines the fourth dimension, time, through the wavy line, which implies spin, or, motion over a duration. (Figure 2)

So, what does it mean to say that Tai Chi embodies the movement of the tai chi symbol? It must, at least in part, be that the motions of Tai Chi generate a dynamic similar to that represented by the tai chi symbol: It must create a ball of motion or action that has the potential to spin around an axis. Planets are large-scale bodies that also spin around an axis, but they spin only in one direction, and their axis is

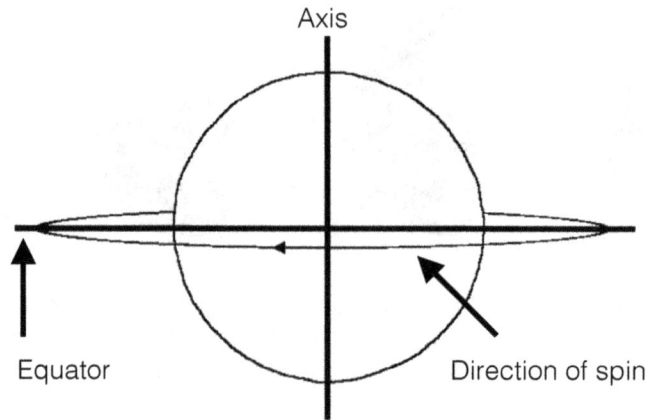

**Figure 3** A planet's axis of spin is 90° to the plane of its equator.

fixed. In addition, a planet's axis is generally stable in relation to the surrounding solar system. Although the axes of many actual planets are not perpendicular to the planet's orbit but are, like Earth's, tilted to one degree or another and might even wobble, for the sake of discussion, I'm referring to an ideal planet with an axis that is at 90° to the plane of its equator and that does not wobble. (Figure 3)

Unlike that of a planet, the axis of the Tai Chi sphere is not fixed in relation to its surroundings, nor must the Tai Chi sphere spin in only one direction. The spinning Tai Chi sphere's axis can shift in relation to its surroundings, allowing the ball to roll in any direction for a specific duration then either stop or rotate to spin in any other direction, dictated only by the will and the limits of human physiology.

The Tai Chi sphere also implies two very different dynamics: the motions of the body's physical movements themselves and the energetic effects that those motions produce. I'll discuss these at length as we go along, but for now, let's briefly consider the energy that forms the substance of this spinning ball. It is called chi. Chi is part of the universal energy spectrum, though Western science has largely ignored this force. Ignoring a thing, however, does not mean it does not exist. (It is important to note here that just as there are words in English that look or sound similar but have very different meanings—be, bee, Bea, for example—so too in other languages. Chi is one such word in Chinese. Used alone, "chi" refers to the subtle energy of living beings and the universe, but this meaning is not what is referenced in the name "Tai

Chi Chuan," which is derived from the nomenclature of the tai chi symbol. In this instance, chi means "ultimate," and the whole term means "grand ultimate fist.")

Every living thing puts out a field of biologically produced energy that surrounds its body. This is a fact that is supported by physiology and physics and that can be subjectively felt through the employment of specialized methods of movement, such as Tai Chi, that have been developed to enhance and strengthen the field's intensity and to increase one's sensitivity to it. I covered the specific ways that the body generates this field in *The Wellspring*, and I'll go into some of that later, but my main purpose in this book is to examine the ways that the physical dynamics of Tai Chi's movements can manipulate the chi field to allow the practitioner to tap into it for health and martial arts purposes.

Martial arts in general teach a series of movements that are functional for self-defense, and Tai Chi is no different in training martial techniques and methodology. But Tai Chi is equally famous for promoting health. This is because Tai Chi teaches a method of movement that not only amplifies and strengthens the flow of chi, but that also becomes ingrained in the practitioner's body and is, over time, incorporated into his or her daily movement patterns. While this method of movement lends the Tai Chi exponent the ability to respond appropriately to a physical attack and, if necessary, to retaliate, arguably more important results are balanced, grounded, and fluid daily movements that constantly enhance one's health. After all, few of us will ever have to fight another person, but all of us will have to battle the vicissitudes of life and the effects of aging.

Ironically, though, the health aspect of Tai Chi is rooted in the art's martial function. Tai Chi was not created to serve as a healthful exercise, and its utility as an exercise and health enhancer is inextricably linked to its operation as a martial art, for the martial aspects of Tai Chi explicitly teach one how to strengthen the chi, open the body to allow it to flow, and then to manipulate it within the body and within external reality.

If this idea of a person creating and using a spinning ball of force or energy is correct, there must be a particular dynamic at work. Different ways of utilizing the ball might explain why the many various styles—Chen, Yang, Hao, Wu, Sun, and others—are somewhat different in appearance, focus, and often utility, yet are all still Tai Chi. In the initial chapters that follow, I will discuss the physical dynamics of the Tai Chi movements and try to analyze how they work and what makes them so effective. Because many of the movements—perhaps most—can be persuasively executed with minimal strength in self-defense applications, then the physical dynamics of the movements alone must be part of the martial equation, with the mobilization of the chi, rather than strength, being the factor that adds power to the force of the movements. Since the physiological structures used in creating and mobilizing chi throughout the body were discussed in *The Wellspring*, they won't be more than touched on here. Instead, in later chapters, I'll look at how chi is transformed into power to bolster martial force.

Understanding Tai Chi's principles and utility has its starting point in two fertile fields. One is the Tai Chi Classics, the corpus of older writings on Tai Chi that have informed Tai Chi study since the earliest of them were supposedly discovered in a Beijing salt shop in the late nineteenth century by Wu Ch'eng-ch'ing, brother of Wu Yu-hsiang, founder of Hao style. Other Classics followed, generated mainly by members of the Chen, Yang, and two Wu families and their disciples. These writings, often couched in metaphor and poetic terminology, contain significant theoretical and philosophical information on the art and bear regular re-reading. As do many of what I call the "neo-classics" such as *Wu Style Tai Chi Chuan* by Wu Kung-cho, and modern classics, such as *The Tao of Tai-Chi Chuan* by Jou Tsung Hwa.

The other field from which I harvested my ideas is the physical side of Tai Chi: the Thirteen Postures. These are, in essence, a codification of the martial principles underlying Tai Chi. They are, again, the sum of the four Cardinal Energies, the four Ordinal Energies, and the Five Stances. It was, in fact, while I was attempting to comprehend what exactly the four Cardinal Energies are that I concluded that while many people could expertly utilize the Cardinal Energies in push hands and fighting, they were all giving a less-than-perfect description of the underlying principles.

It strikes me that these two fields—the mental and the physical—perfectly embody the yin and yang aspects of Tai Chi, and thus form their own Tai Chi sphere of exploration into how Tai Chi works. So let's get that ball rolling, and see where it travels.

# (1) Learning Tai Chi

While most people understand that every movement in Tai-Chi Chuan is circular, they do not usually know that the movements are square as well. For example, we see that the diagram of the Four Directions has a square on the outside, but a circle on the inside. The square and circle are tangent to each other. They represent the outside appearance of the movements Peng, Lu, Chi and An, which form a square at first but later generate an inner circular movement.

—Jou Tsung Hwa[4]

**Tai Chi trains** the practitioner in two forms of energy—physical force and chi power—and as we will see, the gestalt of these two is greater than the sum of their parts. Achieving this gestalt is the core of Tai Chi, and it also is why the process can take years or decades as skill and understanding accrue and grow together. Each person is different and learns and comprehends differently and within different time frames. But then, this isn't really an issue because learning Tai Chi isn't a race. It has no finish line or final goal.

Nor is Tai Chi an achievement, exactly. It's not a case of me becoming better at it than my teachers, or my students becoming better at it than I am. Instead, it's a matter of each one of us constantly striving to become better than we were before. Tai Chi doesn't have an end because it is a process of development that continues as long as one practices and deepens the more one explores its ramifications. For some practitioners, Tai Chi is just a good and interesting exercise; for others, it is a way of life. But for all, it begins with the process of learning to perform a form.

In Tai Chi society, it is said that learning Tai Chi requires three elements: natural ability, a good teacher, and perseverance. Of these, natural ability is the least important, a good teacher is next, and perseverance is the most important. While it is true that if you aren't taught properly, you can miss the mark and never comprehend the essence of Tai Chi, it is even more true that if you don't persevere—practice daily with patience and determination over a period of years—it doesn't matter how good your teacher is or how physically adept you might be: You will never learn Tai Chi. I tell my students that while there are several somewhat physically challenging movements in Tai Chi, such as Snakes Creeps Down, the most difficult movement to do also is the one that is physically easiest to perform. It is Preparation. Even though you are just standing there comfortably, this posture implies the entire form that is to follow. In other words, the most difficult movement is to make yourself step into your Tai Chi space each day and practice the form.

But daily practice doesn't just mean doing the form over and over, like a pianist practicing her scales. It means doing Tai Chi as an integral part of one's daily life—more akin to a physician practicing medicine. It often is noted that there are many people who have faithfully performed Tai Chi for years or even decades yet who are unable to evoke the energies and powers that Tai Chi can impart. What these folks miss are aspects such as bodily awareness, intent, and purpose. These don't come from just going through the motions of the Tai Chi form with your body. They come from attempting to perfect those motions by investing them with practical meaning, both inside your body and out, and studying how that feels to you and observing its effects on others.

So, it is important to understand that the true self-development benefits of Tai Chi—health, spiritual advancement, and so forth—cannot be separated from the art's martial aspect. Tai Chi isn't just waving your arms around in the air in arcane patterns. It is work. When you do Tai Chi, you are performing a series of tasks, each of which involves specific types of body movement and varieties of manipulation of body parts, alignments, and energies. And you should feel like you actually are doing those tasks, but rather than using gross muscular contraction and release to accomplish them, you predominantly use a separate set of physiological structures, coupled with will, attention, and intention. These, in addition to Tai Chi's use of chi and other elements, are what characterize Tai Chi as an "internal" martial art.

If Tai Chi teaches a method of movement that contains martial techniques, it also is a method that uses those martial techniques to increase both the physical (not muscular) force and energetic power of the body. It also teaches one how to become sensitive to that energetic power and to manipulate it in various ways. There are other arts that can teach ways to increase and sensitize one to chi power, such as meditation, but few show a way for chi to freely circulate, not just within the torso, but within the limbs as well, in ways that can have practical, real-world utility. Most of the other methods that can do this include the other internal martial arts, such as Hsing-I and Bagua, among others.

Much is made in the martial arts in general of "lineage." This means learning directly from someone whose personal martial forbearers stand in a long line of practitioners that extends back to the martial art of the Chen family of Henan Province, China. I gave you my modest lineage in the "Preface." What a privilege it would be to learn directly from great masters, but the truth is, most people around the world learn, like I did, primarily from mid-level practitioners. These folks, no less than well-known masters, have a real, if less illustrious, lineage back to the great founding masters, and even if they aren't famous, their forms can be genuine, and their understanding of Tai Chi's underlying principles and utility can be profound.

So, the element of lineage that truly counts most is whether or not the form you learn is genuine and sound: Do its movements adhere to the dynamics ordained by the Thirteen Postures, to the principles established by generation after generation of practitioners, and to the tenets of Tai Chi as laid out in the Tai Chi Classics and other more recent but no less important works on Tai Chi?

Accuracy of form is important for Tai Chi to function properly—martially, energetically, and health-wise—and the reason for that is quite basic: The best teacher of any martial art is the form itself, for any form is a catalog of that art's techniques and methodology. The real key is to learn a solidly functional form from someone who can perform that form accurately and faithfully. If you learn a form that is "real" and then diligently pursue a sincere study of it over time, you will learn real Tai Chi.

I discovered fa jin, for example, on my own, without ever hearing of it or seeing it demonstrated—this was before the advent of personal computers and so was well before the Internet and *YouTube*. It was simply there in the form, and I eventually noticed how I could use some of the movements to send a pulse or wave of energy through my body that could push powerfully or cause a jolting strike. Not knowing it for fa jin, I called it the "Tai Chi bump." I first discovered it in Press and Slant Flying, but later I found it in many places throughout the form, and that, in turn, led me to discover Tai Chi's whipping action and other ways to use the body and internal energy together to accomplish a task.

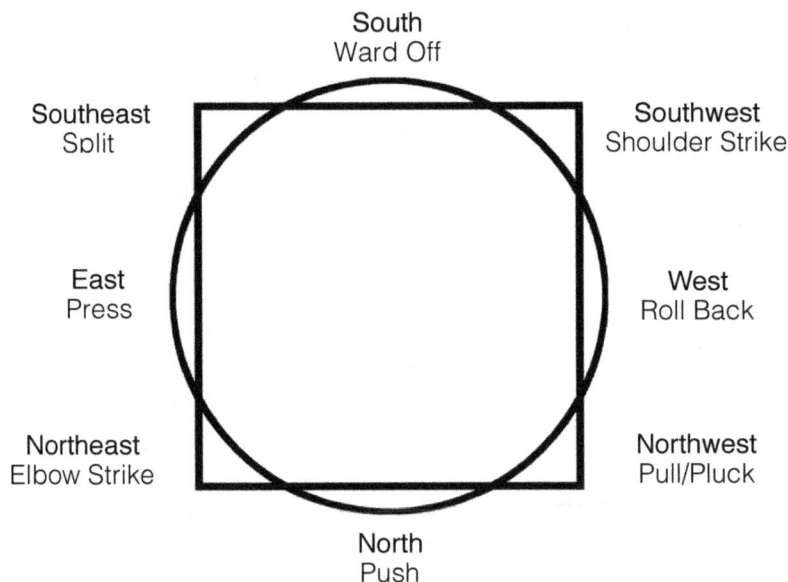

Figure 1.1 Tai Chi movements adhere to two mutually opposing geometrical concepts: the square and the circle. Each of the sides is associated with a direction and a Cardinal Energy, and each of the corners is associated with a direction and an Ordinal Energy. (Note that ancient Chinese maps positioned south at the top.)

An accurate form contains all the secrets; you just have to be observant and study it for its physiological structure, functional possibilities, and energetic states. The benefit of a good teacher is that he or she can teach you an accurate form and then help you discover some of the secrets more rapidly than you otherwise might by working on your own. But it also is true that observation of Tai Chi in action, such as in application videos and movie fight scenes, can serve as a teacher, especially if you have one or more Tai Chi practice partners who enjoy finding ways to use Tai Chi for self-defense.

The point is to discover what truths and possibilities reside in your form and then learn to include them within your practice. By doing this work, you learn to sense your chi, build it, and eventually use it to help generate a wave or pulse of martial force. One significant side effects of this ability is that it teaches one to mobilize the chi, which leads to better health because chi is directly linked to the body's natural healing energies. (See my book *The Wellspring* for a more thorough discussion of this.)

But even if you learn real Tai Chi, don't expect to ever reach some end to the learning process. Tai Chi, no matter which school the practitioner follows, is fractal. The deeper you look, the deeper it goes, and while it may continue to look the same on the outside, it constantly unfolds new levels within—not just of knowledge, but of understanding, awareness, and sensitivity. This is one way the Tai Chi form resembles the tai chi symbol, whose spinning creates a central vortex that opens infinitely into the void of the Tao. The upshot is that once you've learned a Tai Chi form, the work really begins: a lifetime of practice, attention, and observation—in short, perseverance.

Tai Chi movements adhere to two mutually opposing geometrical concepts: the circle and the square. (Figure 1.1) Each of the four Cardinal Energies is identified with its own side of the square, and each of the four Ordinal Energies is identified with a corner—hence their being associated with the cardinal and ordinal compass directions. The square defines the dimensions of the physical world. The circle defines the curving way in which Tai Chi operates within the dimensional physical world. Normally, this is depicted as a circle completely enclosed in a square, but I'm using a diagram that depicts a circle and a square of equal volume. I prefer this figure because, as a martial art, Tai Chi has parallels to the mathematical idea of "squaring the circle," and its inverse, "circling the square": the geometrical challenge of constructing a square with the same area as a given circle, or defining a circle with the same area as a given square.

These tasks were deemed impossible using standard geometrical tools in 1882 when the Lindermann–Weierstrass theorem proved that pi ($\pi$), a necessary element required if one is to accurately determine the area of a circle, is not an algebraic number but rather a transcendental irrational number—a number that recedes into infinity the more you attempt to define it. (Figure 1.2) It is, in short, infinitely deep and thus impossible to accurately pin down. For most purposes, mathematicians usually just cut off the string of numbers at some point and go with the approximation that results.

Tai Chi takes a practical, experiential approach to circling the square, which is evident in the Tai Chi Classics' instruction to "eliminate hollows and projections."

3.14159265358979323846264338327950288419716939937510....

Figure 1.2 Pi, the ratio of a circle's circumference to its diameter, is a fraction whose decimal representation never ends. Here, it is calculated to the 50th decimal place.

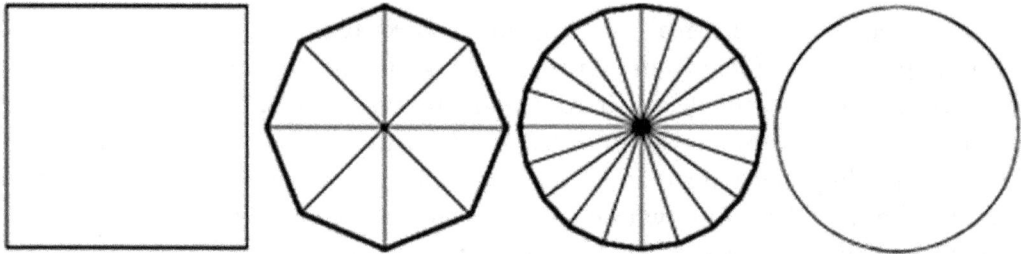

**Figure 1.3** Continually adding sides to a square can simulate roundness, but the resulting figure will never actually be round. Left to right: a square, an octagon (eight sides), an icosagan (20 sides), and a megagon (one million sides). Even if drawn at the size of the Earth, a megagon would be very difficult to distinguish from a circle, but it is still made up of straight lines.

This means to find places in your form where your movements lose continuity or are jerky or too angular, all of which break the smooth and conjoined flow of both physical movement and energy transfer. You can solve the problem by working to bridge the gaps, smooth out the jerkiness, and hone down the projections, so to speak. In this sense, the rounding of the Tai Chi movements can be likened to a geometric figure to which you constantly add new facets over time. The more facets you add, the rounder the figure becomes. While it is true that you can never actually circle the square by this method—even if you add facets infinitely, you will never produce a figure that is truly round—you can make your movements sufficiently rounded for most practical purposes. (Figure 1.3)

True roundness from squareness and true squareness from roundness are technically impossible transitions. But in the pages that follow, we'll see how Tai Chi is an art that trains the body and will to make that magical leap from square to circle then back again. We'll also see how the transformations from the round to the square and back to the round combine with other bodily dynamics to give Tai Chi its legendary force and power.

# ② The Thirteen Postures

T'ai-chi, in its round aspect, whether moving in or out, up or down, left or right never leaves the circle. T'ai-chi, in its square aspect, whether in or out, up or down, left or right never leaves the square. The circle is for issuing or entering; the square is for advancing or retreating. There is a constant back and forth movement from the square to the circle. The square is for opening and expanding and the circle is for closing and contracting.

—Yang family manuscript[5]

**As mentioned earlier,** Tai Chi was originally called, among other things, the Thirteen Postures. The number thirteen refers to the sum of Tai Chi's four Cardinal (principal) Energies, four Ordinal (ancillary) Energies, and Five Stances (the five directions of movement). The Cardinal and Ordinal Energies often are lumped together under the term the "Eight Gates." The Thirteen Postures are at the core of Tai Chi's martial utility and its health-promoting aspects. Many Tai Chi philosophers have linked the Thirteen Postures or their parts to, among other ideas, the five Chinese elements, the compass directions, and the eight trigrams of the *I Ching* or through affinity/antagonism. A discussion of these other correspondences is beyond the scope of this book, which will, instead, focus on the physical and energy dynamics of Tai Chi, beginning with the Thirteen Postures.

The illustrations on the final pages of this section show each of the Thirteen

Postures in one of the basic Tai Chi movements commonly associated with that posture. Of course, these are just examples since most of the movements in a Tai Chi form demonstrate one or more aspects and/or combinations of the Thirteen Postures. In general, Tai Chi practitioners traditionally refer to the Thirteen Postures, and particularly the Eight Gates, as techniques and/or applications. See this, for example, from the Tai Chi Classics:

> Ward-off is in the two arms.
> Roll-back is in the palms.
> Press is in the back of the hand.
> Push is in the waist.
> Pull-down is in the fingers.
> Split is in the two forearms.
> Elbow-stroke involves bending the limbs.
> Shoulder-stroke employs shoulder against chest.[6]

But I have a problem with defining the Eight Gates as techniques or applications. If we, as Tai Chi exponents, are going to refer to these eight elements as "energies," then we should look at them in that light to discover their specific characteristics and functions *as* unique expressions of energy. Moreover, the descriptions normally given to the four Cardinal Energies generally lack the concept of their opposites. You can see this with Ward Off, which is usually described as a yang movement, or Roll Back, which is described as a yin one. Again, if an art is to be called Tai Chi, then it must adhere to the precepts of the tai chi symbol and equally exhibit yin and yang characteristics throughout.

The purpose of the first part of this book is to suggest a different way to look at the Thirteen Postures—especially the Eight Gates—than is generally used and that, while not being traditional, does not, I believe, violate the principles traditionally ascribed to Tai Chi. Instead of beginning with the Eight Gates, though, I'm going to start the discussion with the Five Stances. After all, performing Tai Chi well requires a firm foundation.

# The Thirteen Postures

(Chinese names for the Cardinal and Ordinal Energies are given in italics following the English term.)

## The Five Stances

(Five Steps, Five Elements)

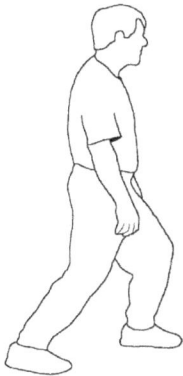

**Step Forward**
Advance
Metal: Gives birth to water
and destroys wood

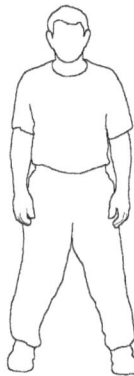

**Central Equilibrium**
A rooting stance that
remains centered
Earth: Gives birth to metal
and destroys water

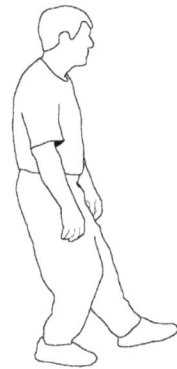

**Step Backward**
Retreat
Wood: Gives birth to fire
and destroys earth

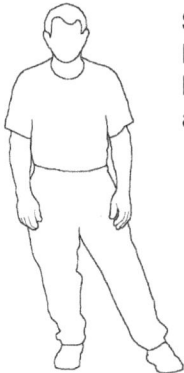

**Step Right**
Moving to the right
Fire: Gives birth to earth
and destroys metal

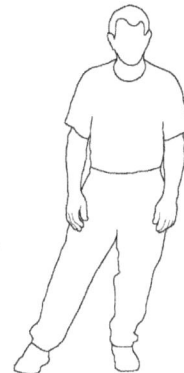

**Step Left**
Moving to the left
Water: Gives birth to wood
and destroys fire

# The Eight Gates

## The Four Cardinal Energies
(Principal Energies, Cardinal Directions)

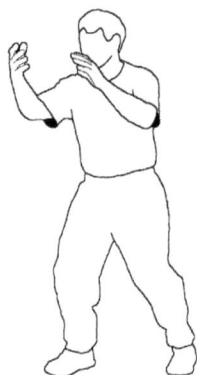

**Ward Off**
(Peng, heaven, south)
An outward and upward
expansion of energy

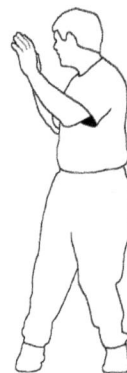

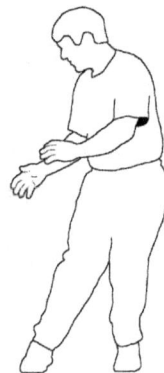

**Roll Back**
(Lu, earth, west)
An inward-receiving energy that
moves incoming force back
and to the side, high or low

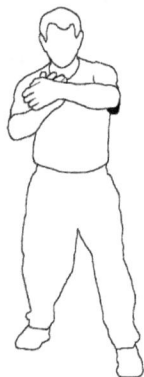

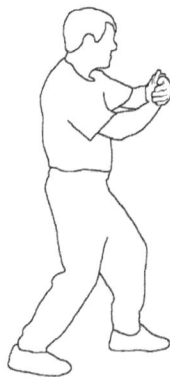

**Press**
(Ji, water, east)
An outward-moving energy of
compression or squeezing

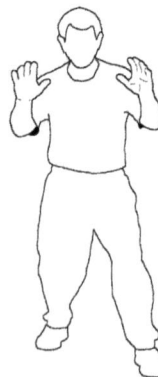

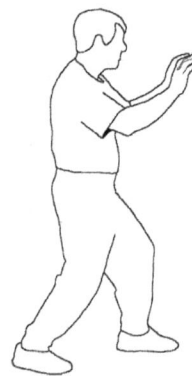

**Push**
(An, fire, north)
An outward- or
downward-moving energy

# The Four Ordinal Energies
(Ancillary Energies, Ordinal Directions)

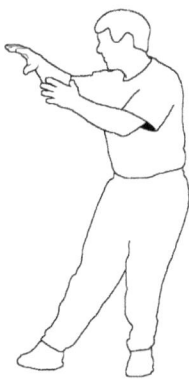

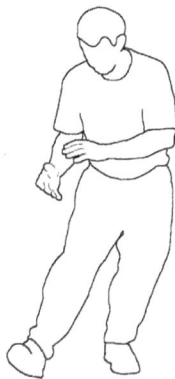

**Pull / Pluck**
(Cai, wind, northwest)
A grabbing and pulling
energy, high or low

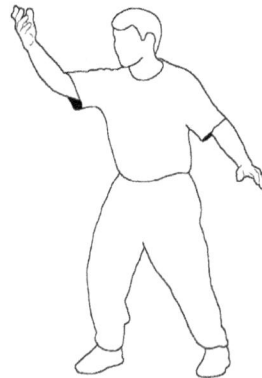

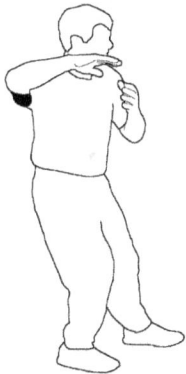

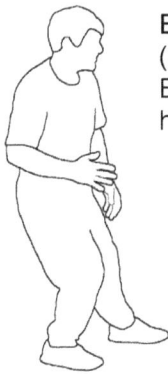

**Elbow Strike**
(Zhou, lake, northeast)
Elbow striking energy,
high or low

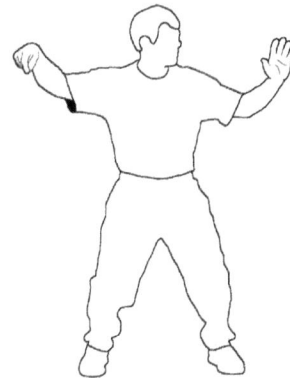

**Split**
(Lie, thunder, southeast)
An energy that moves
apart from a center

**Shoulder Strike**
(Kao, mountain, southwest)
Full-body striking energy

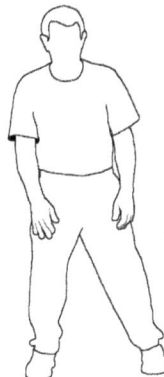

# The Five Stances

**The Five Stances** are, at their most basic, simply the directions in which one can move, issue power, or avoid incoming force. They are: Step Forward, Step Backward, Step Right, Step Left, and Central Equilibrium. On the surface, they might seem obvious: You can move forward and backward, right and left, and by extension, toward any intermediate direction—any angle between forward and right, for example. You also can stand still. (Figure 2.14) Step Forward, which is sometimes referred to as Bow Stance, and Step Backward, which is sometimes referred to as Sitting Stance, both exhibit a critical alignment: The nose, knee, and toes of the

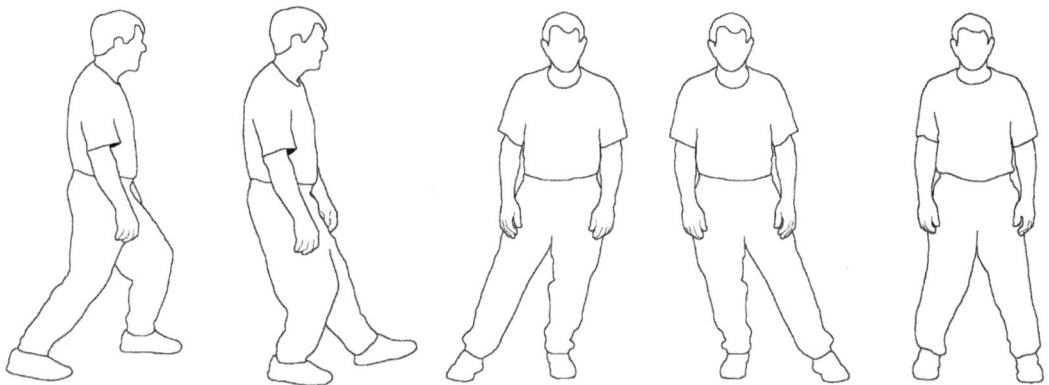

Figure 2.14 The Five Stances (left to right): Step Forward, Step Backward, Step Left, Step Right, and Central Equilibrium.

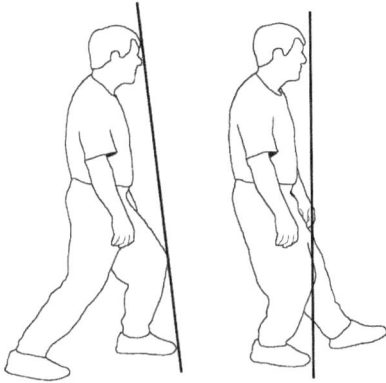

Figure 2.15 Whether in Bow Stance or Sitting Stance, the nose and knee and toes of the weighted leg should line up.

weighted leg should all line up. (Figure 2.15) This ensures a stable stance that is not over-extended, insufficiently extended, or leaning backward, but that goes straight down into the root of the weighted leg.

Step Forward and Step Backward initiate the idea of yang (force) and yin (yielding) through body movements. They also demonstrate Tai Chi's two most basic tactics: advance to issue force and power for attack, and retreat to ab-sorb or redirect force and power for defense. Step Forward and Step Backward also suggest a stable and balanced method of walking ei-ther forward or backward. (Figure 2.16) As the Classics say, "Walk like a cat."

Things get stickier with Step Left and Step Right, so let's look at those a little more close-ly. At the basic level, one can simply shift one's weight to one side or the other, and in this respect, they are like a Sitting Stance, done to one side or the other, that uti-lizes the same nose-knee-toes alignment noted above. (Figure 2.17) Tactically, this is a basic evasion movement: simply move to one side or the other to get out of the

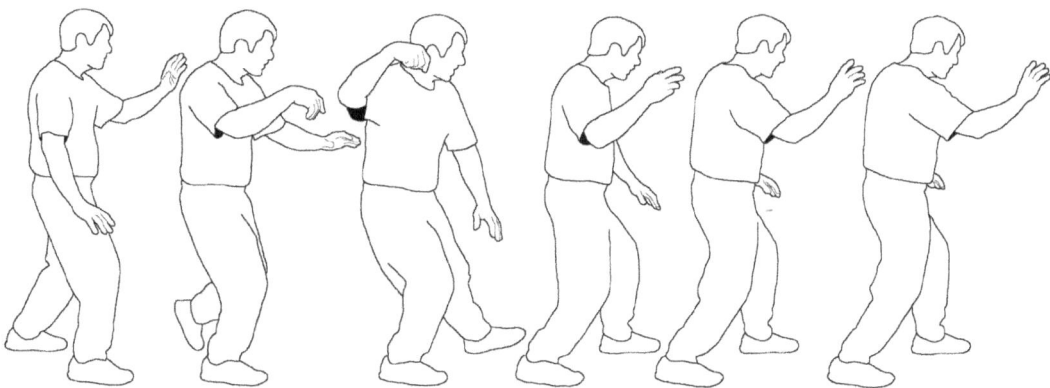

Figure 2.16 Step Forward implies an advancing walking pattern—shown here with Brush Knee Twist Step. Reversing the walking pattern produces a retreat, as with Mon-key Moving Backward.

way of an incoming force. This method is useful up to a point, but it might not actually be the quickest or most effective way to get out of the line of fire. The way toward that is by thinking of these two stances as Look Left and Look Right, which is what some people call them. (Figure 2.18)

Looking is a lot different than shifting. Because turning the head to look to either side entails a certain amount of twisting around the spine, thinking of these stances as Looking Left and Looking Right adds awareness of this central axis —or Central Equilibrium—to the critical Tai Chi physical ideal of maintaining a balanced posture that is capable of turning and moving rapidly. (Figure 2.19) As the Tai Chi Classics say: "Stand like a balance, move like a wheel." The "balance" is Central Equilibrium, around which the wheel of the waist turns.

But as Tai Chi exponents know, Central Equilibrium is just the beginning because Tai Chi's martial attacks and defense are based on the solid platform of a stable stance that has most of the weight rooted on one leg. And Tai Chi exponents also know that, as the awareness goes, so too goes the body. According to the Tai Chi Classics, Tai Chi

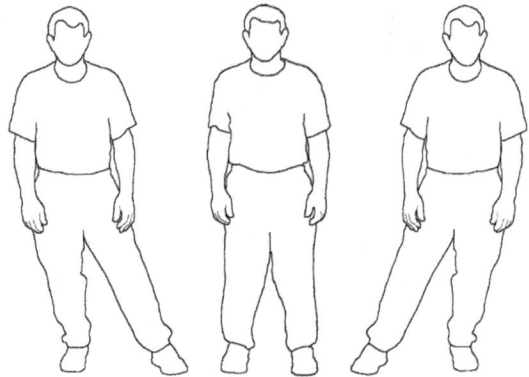

Figure 2.17 Stepping sideways or shifting the weight is one of the simplest ways to avoid an incoming force.

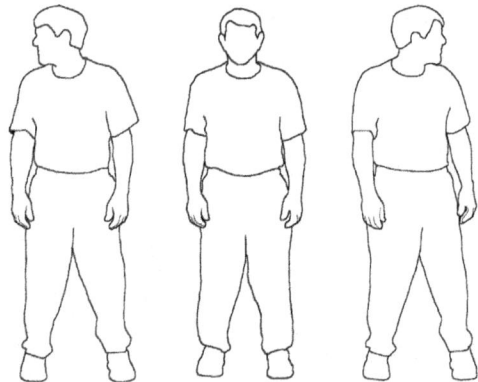

Figure 2.18 Twisting the head to look in either direction emphasizes Tai Chi's posture of Central Equilibrium because the head twists on the central ridgepole of the spine.

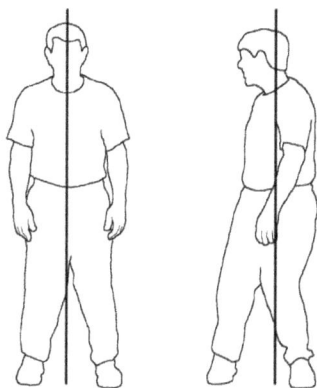

Figure 2.19 The central axis emphasizes rotation around the body's core.

movements are "initiated by the legs, directed by the waist, transmitted by the torso and arms, and expressed in the hands." Think of standing in Central Equilibrium, then looking to one side or the other. If you adhere to the Classics' admonition to initiate movement from the legs and direct it with the waist, then you can't simply turn your head and/or shoulders to look right or left. You also must rotate your waist—the "wheel."

This causes your torso to turn in the appropriate direction, but once it does, another Tai Chi rule comes into play, telling you to avoid committing the defect of double-weighting. Double-weighting and some of the alternate ways of looking at it will be discussed at various points later, so for now, suffice it to say that, at its most basic, double-weighting is placing your weight too evenly on both feet.

For this reason, if you look sideways in one direction, you have to shift your weight to the opposite leg as you turn so that you won't be double-weighted. You could shift onto the leg closest to your attacker, but you wouldn't want to lean into the incoming force. Instead, you sit back, away from the incoming force. Because of the waist turn, this sitting back naturally assumes a circular motion. (Figure 2.20) From there, you can continue the backward circling by sinking your weight onto the weighted leg. This will allow you to lead the incoming force to the side, rebound it, or swallow it.

So if you look in a direction, your Tai Chi-trained body will automatically tend to turn itself, also, away from the direction in which you are looking, causing your torso to turn until your navel points in the same direction as you face: at your opponent. Now these two stances become Look Left to Move Right and Look Right to Move Left, as they are sometimes called. In them, the idea of going side-to-side finds another layer of complexity in terms of the way the body might move and of Tai Chi's martial tactics.

While just shifting to the right or left is essentially a linear, unidirectional movement—and a yang, or forceful, action—turning and sitting are both yielding actions, thus adding the dimension of yin to the yang of simply moving to the left or right. Unlike the linear avoidance of stepping sideways or leaning to one side or the other, Looking Left to Move Right and Looking Right to Move Left train one in what might be called a shift-twist-sink retreat—an evasion that moves away, turns, and sinks all at the same time. Yielding to an incoming force simultaneously in three different dimensions greatly magnifies the retreat's speed and effective distance. Plus, it leaves the body in a well-balanced position for further retreat or for a counter-attack. We'll look at yielding in more detail later when we discuss the Cardinal Energy of Roll Back.

Thinking of these two side stances in this more complex way shows that they embody another maxim from the Tai Chi Classics: "In order to move in any direction, one must first move, however slightly, in the opposite direction." Tai Chi, after all, adheres closely to the laws of physics—in this case Newton's third law: "For every action, there is an equal and opposite reaction."

Central Equilibrium emphasizes the practitioner's central axis, or the central core of the body, but the idea of Central Equilibrium is a little more complex than just rotating around your core because, as the movements of the shift-twist-sink retreat show, there are two other vertical axes: one on each side of your body. They run through the heel, hip, and shoulder. (Figure 2.21)

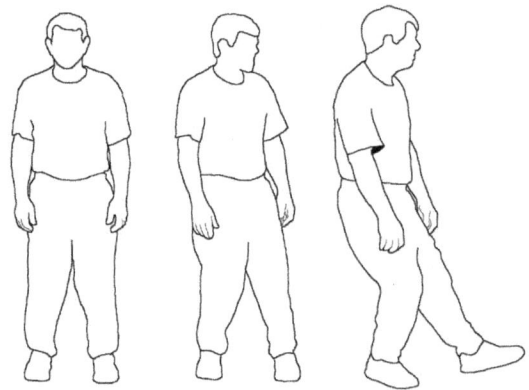

Figure 2.20 Looking Left to Move Right adds sitting and turning to the basic linear movement of a simple Step Right, twisting one away from incoming force.

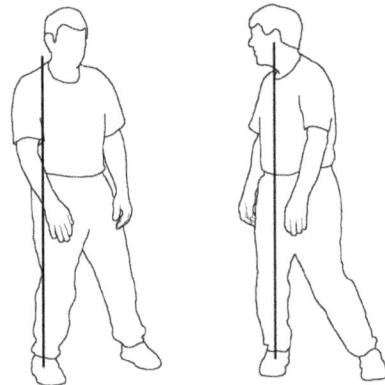

Figure 2.21 The axes on each side of the body allow rotation around each side. The right axis is shown here.

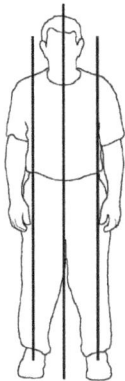

Figure 2.22
The three ver-
tical axes

So Look Left to Move Right and Look Right to Move Left don't just demonstrate movement toward either of those directions; they illustrate the three axes around which the body twists and turns to accomplish its movements. (Figure 2.22) This, in turn, leads to the basic Tai Chi idea of shifting your weight back and forth from leg to leg, with the ability to rotate around any one of the three axes or around two or three of them in sequence. And if you rotate your waist while you shift back and forth, you automatically employ a circling of your hips in a figure-eight pattern as your legs push your body weight from one side to the other and back again. This lends the ability to shift your weight, turn, or otherwise move without halting the momentum of your hips and waist. (Figure 2.23)

This figure-eight pattern of hip movement is critical to Tai Chi's operation, and I'll look at it in more detail later. For now, it's enough to point out that some Tai Chi movements rotate principally around the central axis of the spine—Single Whip, for example. Others rotate around one or the other side axis—Parry and Punch, for example. And yet others use a sequential rotation of all three vertical axes, from right to left or in the opposite direction—Wave Hands Like Clouds, for example. However, Central Equilibrium is the most important vertical axis. It defines the body's center of rotation, and it is the axis most used. When you use one of the side vertical axes, you always get there from Central Equilibrium, and it is to Central Equilibrium that you always return.

We can see that Tai Chi deserves the name of Grand Ultimate Fist if the essence of the art is built into the stances alone. But there's more to come. The three vertical axes are important to understand the Four Cardinal Energies and the ways they function physically and energetically, and we'll look at those next.

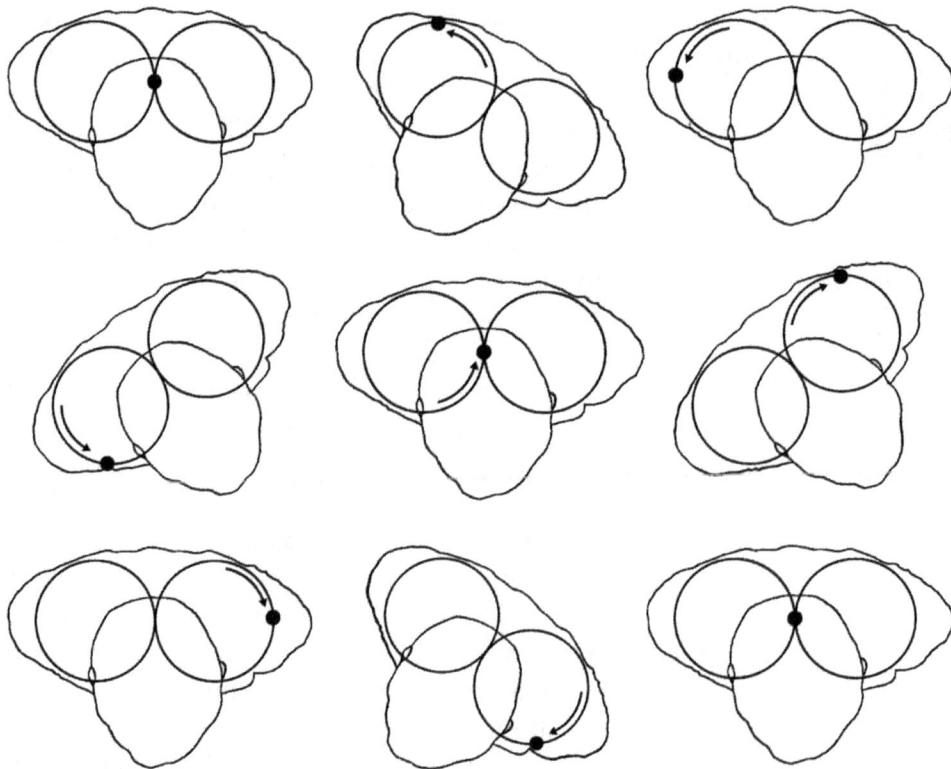

Figure 2.23 If you rotate your waist while you shift your weight back and forth between the legs, you automatically employ a circling your hips in a figure-eight pattern. This lends the ability to shift your weight, turn, or otherwise move without halting the momentum of your hips and waist. The dot represents the point where the weight is greatest, and the arrow indicates the direction of circling. This figure shows circling through the figure-eight in one direction, but you also can circle it in the other direction.

# The Cardinal Energies

**The four Cardinal** Energies often are equated with the types of forces the Tai Chi exponent utilizes for self-defense. In reality, it is actually the same energy—usually called Peng—but it is directed in each of four very different ways, each of which is embodied in a Cardinal Energy. The Cardinal Energies are (Figure 2.24):

1. Ward Off (Peng, heaven, south): An outward and upward expansion of energy
2. Roll Back (Lu, earth, west): An inward-receiving energy that diverts incoming energy to the side and back.
3. Press (Ji, water, east): An outward-moving energy of compression or squeezing
4. Push (An, fire, north): A forward- or downward-moving energy

While the Cardinal Energies might have relatively pure and full expressions within the form, in practical terms, they are only rarely expressed that way. Most often, they are found in combination with one or more of the other Cardinal Energies, and usually they are expressed within only a small portion of the full range of which they are capable. Usually, they are listed in the order given above, but this order, particularly in the Yang style, refers to a possible sequence of defenses and attacks, and as I said earlier, I'm trying to approach the matter from the standpoint of how each Cardinal Energy operates in a distinctive way to express internal force and energy, rather than from the standpoint of its specific martial applications. So I

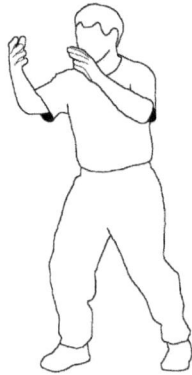

**Ward Off**
(Peng, heaven, south)
An outward and upward
expansion of energy

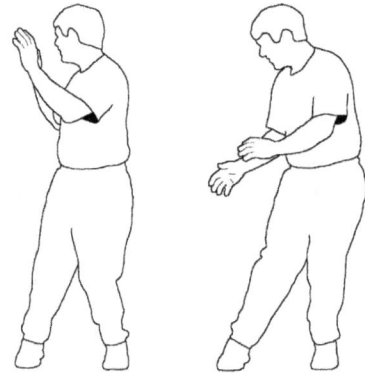

**Roll Back**
(Lu, earth, west)
An inward- receiving energy
that moves incoming force
back and to the side

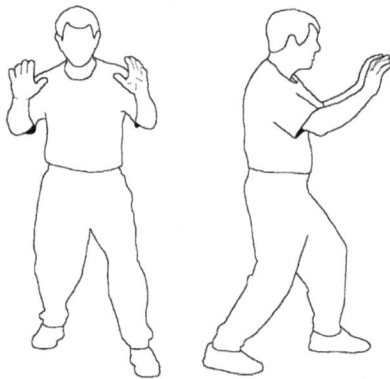

**Push**
(An, fire, north)
An outward- or downward-
moving energy

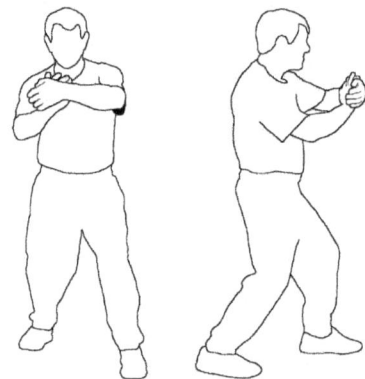

**Press**
(Ji, water, east)
An outward-moving energy
of compression or squeezing

Figure 2.24 The Four Cardinal Energies (cardinal directions).

had to scrap any preconceptions born of possible usage and focus on the functionally different characteristics of each of them.

I felt I had a good grasp of the basic martial functions of the Cardinal Energies as performed in the form of Tai Chi that I do—a modified version of Northern Wu Style—but one particular element continued to puzzle me: Push. On the surface, this might seem to be the simplest of the Cardinal Energies: You push from your root—usually using the back leg—and let the force of the push move as a muscular and energetic wave up your leg, through your waist, torso, and arms, then to the hands. But an often-used description of Push is that it is a backward and downward moving energy. Okay, I could feel how the force and energy move down into the feet, but in the form I do, the force and energy then surge up the legs, through the waist and torso, and finally, through the arms and into the hands—still a forward and outward moving energy. How could it be both forward and outward, and backward and downward?

When I began doing Tai Chi in the late 1970s, there weren't a lot of resources available to the practitioner. There were probably fewer than two dozen books on the subject in English, a bare handful of which presented more than a cursory history of the art and often-inadequate instructions describing how to do a particular form. And there was precious little visual material. Consumer video tape players had been on the market for less than five years, and the number of Tai Chi videos was practically nonexistent, and the few out there tended to be expensive. And of course, the personal computer had yet to be invented, so the Internet and YouTube weren't even glimmers on the horizon. Since then, the number of good to excellent books on Tai Chi have proliferated, and maybe more important, so have the number of videos. After all, Tai Chi is a dynamic art. Much can be said about it with words, but visual demonstrations of physical movements are invaluable, whether for form instruction or for self-defense applications.

So when in recent years I began wondering about Push, I consulted my Tai Chi library and read what I could find there on the Thirteen Postures—in particular, the four Cardinal Energies. Then I went online and read some more. Next I looked at online videos. What I found made me think I'd time traveled back to the late 1970s because of the dearth of material. Despite showing some expert practitioners ably demonstrating the Thirteen Postures via their functionality, most of the mere handful of videos on the subject simply reiterated what the written literature said about the energies: Ward Off is an upward and outward energy, Roll Back diverts incoming energy to the side and back, Press is a compressive energy, and Push is either a downward- or outward-moving energy. The problem remained, for the Cardinal Energies were always described in terms of martial techniques rather than as discreet energies with functionally different characteristics.

Not only was my question about Push unanswered, but I discovered I'd stumbled on a new line of inquiry. Each of the four Cardinal Energies usually was associated with a yang or yin force, and while I could feel those in my body when I practiced, I believed that thinking of the Cardinal Energies as techniques rather than energies severely limited the potential range of that energy's expression. Tai Chi is Tai Chi precisely because it plays the entire Tai Chi sphere of yang and yin forces, both forces working together as a unified whole. Describing Press as a yang force or Roll Back as a yin one seemed to leave out half the equation, and as Tai Chi practitioners know, you simply can't do that in Tai Chi or your practice is faulty and incomplete. And to compound matters, there were many movements that don't seem readily identifiable as using any one of the four principal energies as they are traditionally described. On the surface, for example, Brush Knee Twist Step and Golden Cock Stands on One Leg, both of which are very common to most Tai Chi forms, don't obviously use any one of them.

I realized I'd have to try to analyze the Cardinal Energies for myself, attempting to understand them through what was being defined by the Tai Chi form in terms of physical and energy dynamics, all the while, taking into account the yang and yin aspects of each. My first goal was to define each of the Cardinal Energies in its purest, fullest expression, and next, I wanted to understand how each of those pure forms could be altered to express martial utility. I'll pursue that first goal in this chapter and the other aspects in the chapters that follow, but for now, I knew that my starting point had to be the Tai Chi sphere because the sphere is the core of the practice. But I also had to start with Push because, though it should have been the easiest energy to understand, it seemed to be the one I comprehended the least.

# Push

**Why is Push** considered by some to be a downward pulling energy and by others an outward expelling energy? Once I really thought about it, the answer came readily enough, thanks to the concept of the Tai Chi sphere.

Consider the sphere to be a ball in front of your body. This ball's maximum diameter is about the distance from the top of your head to your groin, and it can be as small as a pea. (Figure 2.25) Most commonly, its diameter is about the distance from your shoulders to your tantien. You can loosely hold this ball between your palms and rotate it side to side. (Figure 2.26) (Note that in this and all subsequent illustrations, I'm using the tai chi symbol to indicate rotation of the Tai Chi sphere. The direction of rotation is always toward the head of the yang, or white, portion of the symbol. The moment when the direction of rotation reverses is indicated by a blank symbol.)

Well, if you can rotate the Tai Chi sphere like this, you also can rotate it in other directions. So it was beginning to dawn on

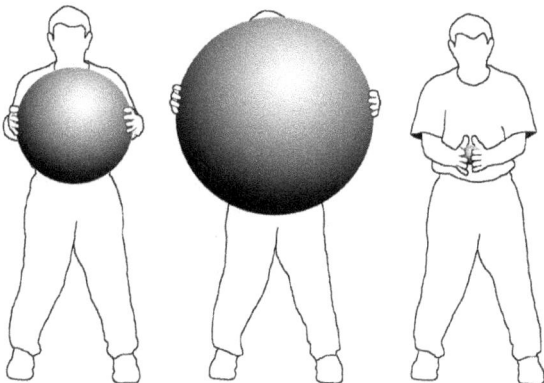

**Figure 2.25** The Tai Chi sphere can be played at various diameters.

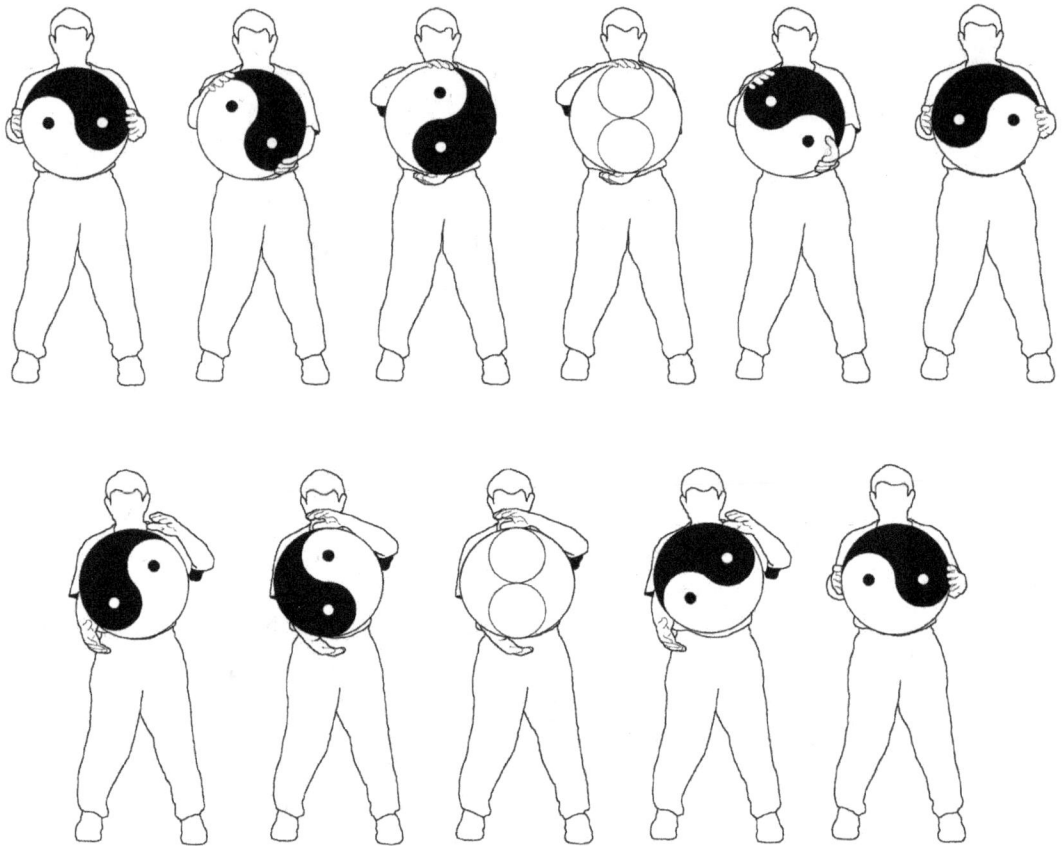

**Figure 2.26** The basic Tai Chi manipulation is to roll the Tai Chi sphere from side to side. The spheres with blank double fish indicate the moment when the energy switches polarity and the ball starts rolling in the opposite direction.

me how to see beyond the technique of Push—to push someone over backward or pull them straight down in front of you—and to see it as an energy that operates in a certain way. Push is a simply rolling the Tai Chi sphere straight forward or straight backward directly in front of the body. (Figure 2.27) Rolling it forward and downward over the top then backward and upward from under the bottom would be the yang aspect, while rolling it backward and downward from over the top then forward and upward from under the bottom would be the yin aspect. Though the impetus for Push can come from both feet at the same time, it usually emanates from one foot or the other. But in any case, Push primarily utilizes Central Equilibrium, or the central core, in combination with either Step Forward or Step Backward.

No matter which direction you spin a ball, a unidirectional rotation around the perimeter of the sphere tends to emphasize the sphere's equator, which spins at right angles to the line of its axis. The equator is where the sphere's spinning force is focused and thus is at its greatest, both in terms of force and reach. (Figure 2.28) Paying attention to the equator tends to de-emphasize the sphere's dimensionality, flattening it into a rotating disk. As often as not, it is this equatorial circumference, rather than the sphere as a whole, that the Tai Chi player employs when expressing any given Cardinal Energy in its purest form.

However, even if the player concentrates on the circumference, the flattening effect does not diminish the force of the whole sphere, for the sphere still exists, lending its entire mass to the focal point. Nor does it negate the three-dimensional nature of the sphere, which still exists even if you're only paying attention to the equator. This is most evident in the fact that you can rotate the angle of sphere's axis at will and thus change the angle and direction of the rotation of its equator. Armed with this idea, I attacked the other three Cardinal Energies.

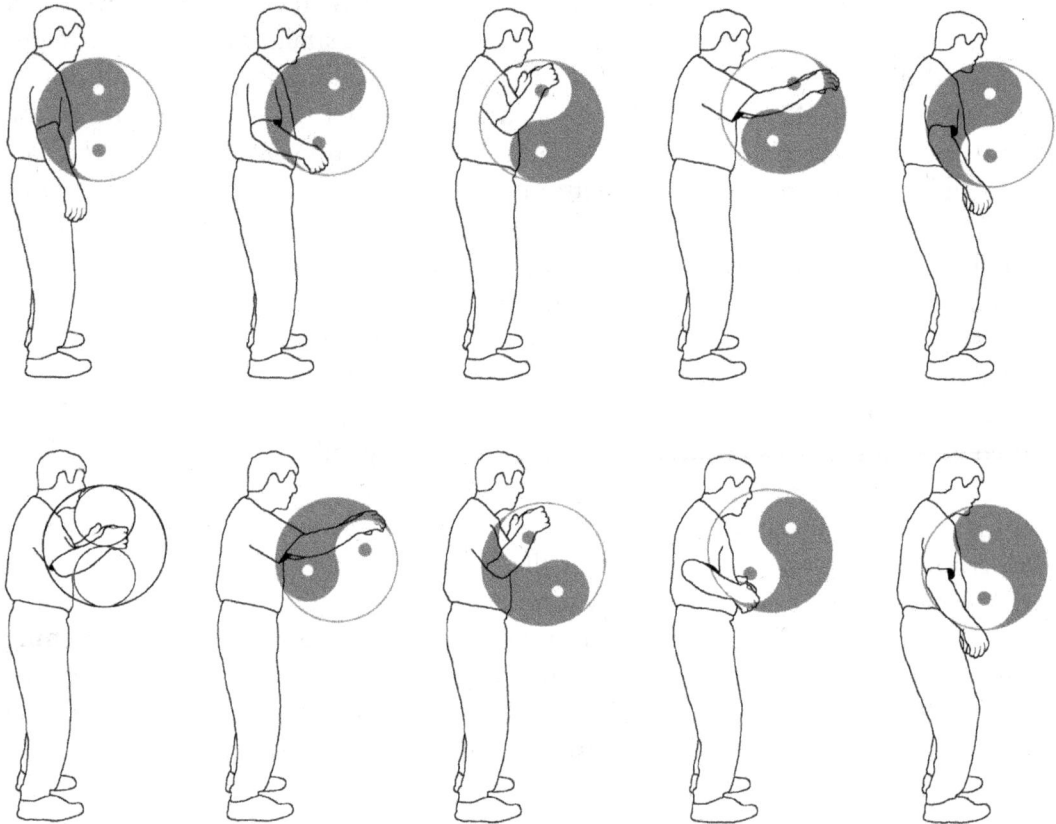

Figure 2.27 The Push ball can be rolled forward and over the top then backward from underneath (top row) or backward over the top then forward from underneath (bottom row). The key is that it rolls straight forward or backward directly in front of the body. The blank symbol is when the energy changes direction.

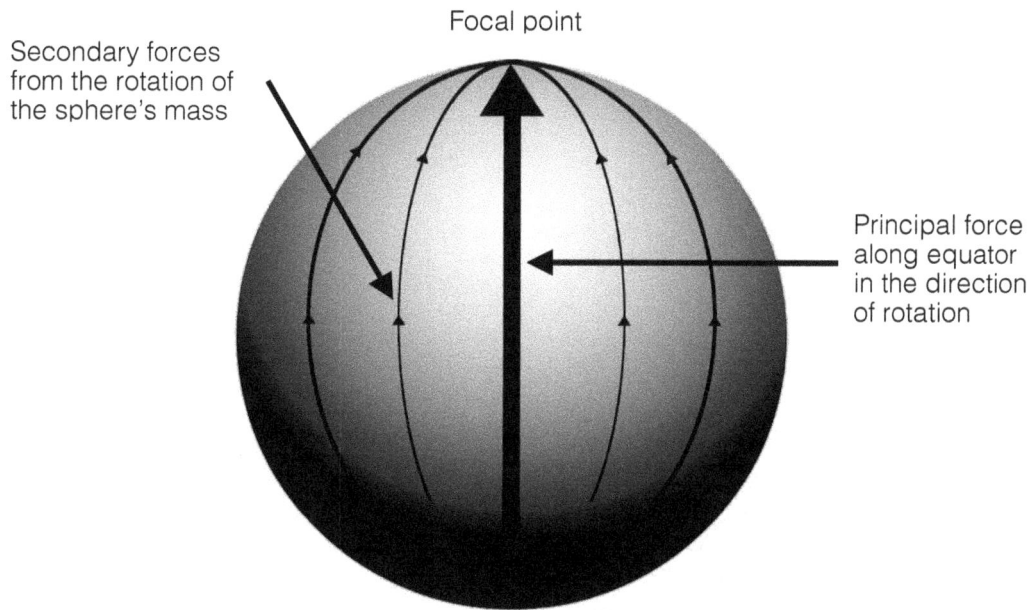

Focal point

Secondary forces
from the rotation of
the sphere's mass

Principal force
along equator
in the direction
of rotation

**Figure 2.28** The force of a rotating sphere is most powerful in the direction of rotation along its equator, but the entire mass of the sphere also rotates in the same direction, adding its inertial power and weight to the focal point.

# Ward Off

**Ward Off, as** a technique, is generally considered to be an upward- and outward-welling energy and also a yang movement because, in part, it can bump off incoming energy in one direction or another. (Figure 2.29) But as I extrapolated from the pure sphere for Push, I saw that Ward Off also employs the sphere, the only difference being the direction of rotation. Push rotates the sphere straight forward and straight backward in front of the body, but Ward Off rotates it diagonally across the body.

When looking at Ward Off's physical movements, you can see how they propel this diagonal rotation: The impetus for Ward Off energy moves upward from the foot and through the leg of one side, then it is directed by the waist across the torso and into the arm and hand on the opposite side from the leg that generated the energy.

In essence, the body is rotating and shifting through all three vertical axes in sequence, either from left to right, or in the opposite direction, and either forward or backward. This causes the circle that is generated at the sphere's equator to rotate diagonally across the body. (Figure 2.30)

Although Ward Off is usually thought of as being a yang energy, as with Push, Ward Off has its yin aspect. If you rotate the circle forward, either from the top or the bottom, the energy is yang, but if you rotate it backward, either from the top or bottom, it is yin. The former lends

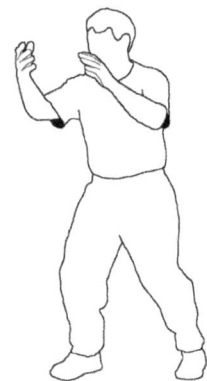

Figure 2.29 Ward Off as a technique.

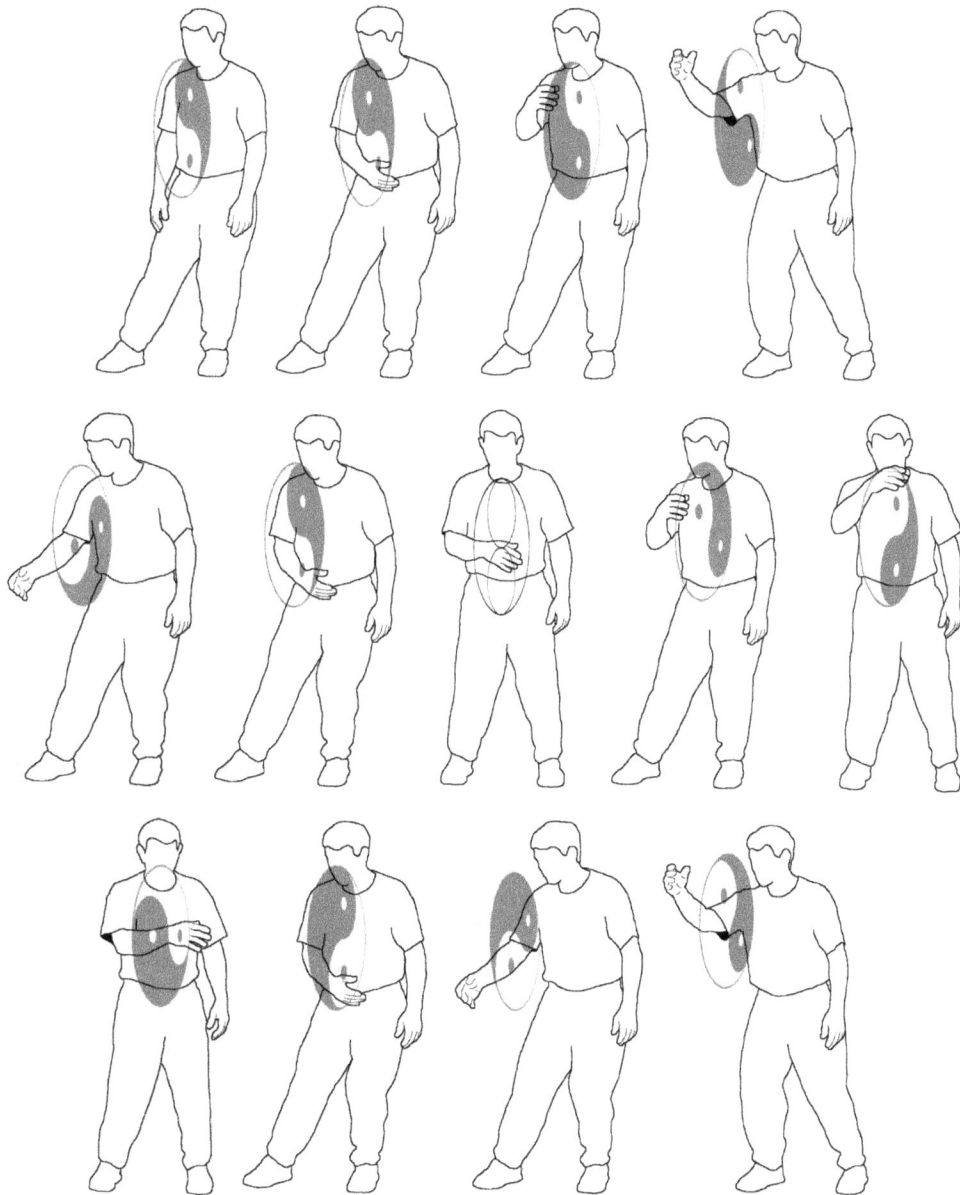

Figure 2.30 The Ward Off energy sphere rotates diagonally across the body. The energy begins in one leg, transfers to the opposite arm, then returns to the original leg. The sphere with blank double fish indicates the moment when the ball starts rolling in the opposite direction.

itself to the usually seen function of using Ward Off as a sort of pneumatic force that can repel or strike, but the latter more easily ties in when it is used with, for example, Roll Back, to power the Ordinal Energy of Pull/Pluck, which would be a yin usage.

Gothic cathedrals ... often include essential elements from the mandala symbolism (that is, the squaring of the circle, through a geometrical diagram combining the square and the circle, usually linked through the octagon as an intermediate step).

—J. E. Cirlot[7]

# Roll Back

**As a technique,** Roll Back is usually considered to be a yielding, or yin, movement because it turns the body away from incoming force. (Figure 2.31) However, it also contains a yang component because, if one side turns away, the other side automatically moves forward at the same time. In addition, Roll Back often cocks the body for a forward movement or other yang follow up. Roll Back was the easiest for me to comprehend as an energy. If Push rolls the sphere/circle straight forward and straight backward, and Ward Off rolls it diagonally across the body, either left to right or vice versa, then Roll Back, in its purest form, repositions the ball to center on the body's corfe and rotates it laterally around that central axis. (Figure 2.32) But it also can, if you shift your body to either the left or right, rotate around the vertical axis on either side. (Figure 2.33)

The arms can come into play in Roll Back at any of three main levels: shoulder height, torso height, and hip height. A maneuver like Wave Hands Like Clouds utilizes Roll Back around all three axes in a smooth sequence from side to side. (Figure 2.34)

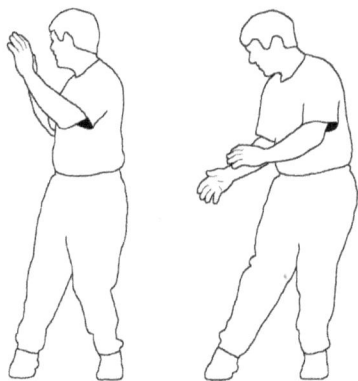

Figure 2.31 Roll Back as techniques.

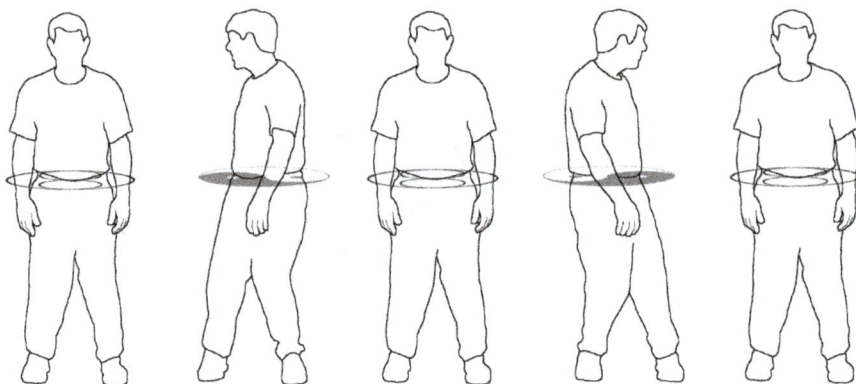

**Figure 2.32** In Roll Back, the Tai Chi sphere rotates backward or forward around the central axis.

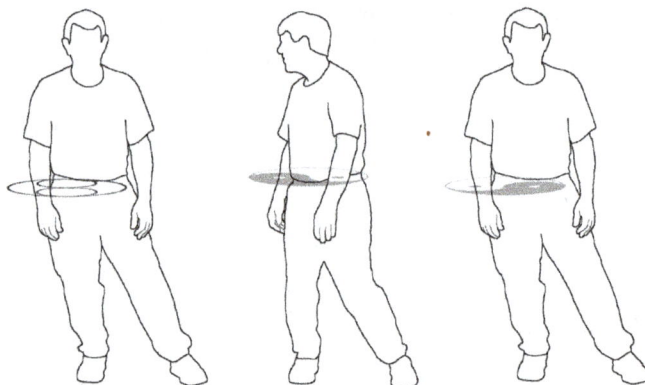

**Figure 2.33** Roll Back also can rotate around either of the side vertical axes. Roll Back around the right axis is illustrated.

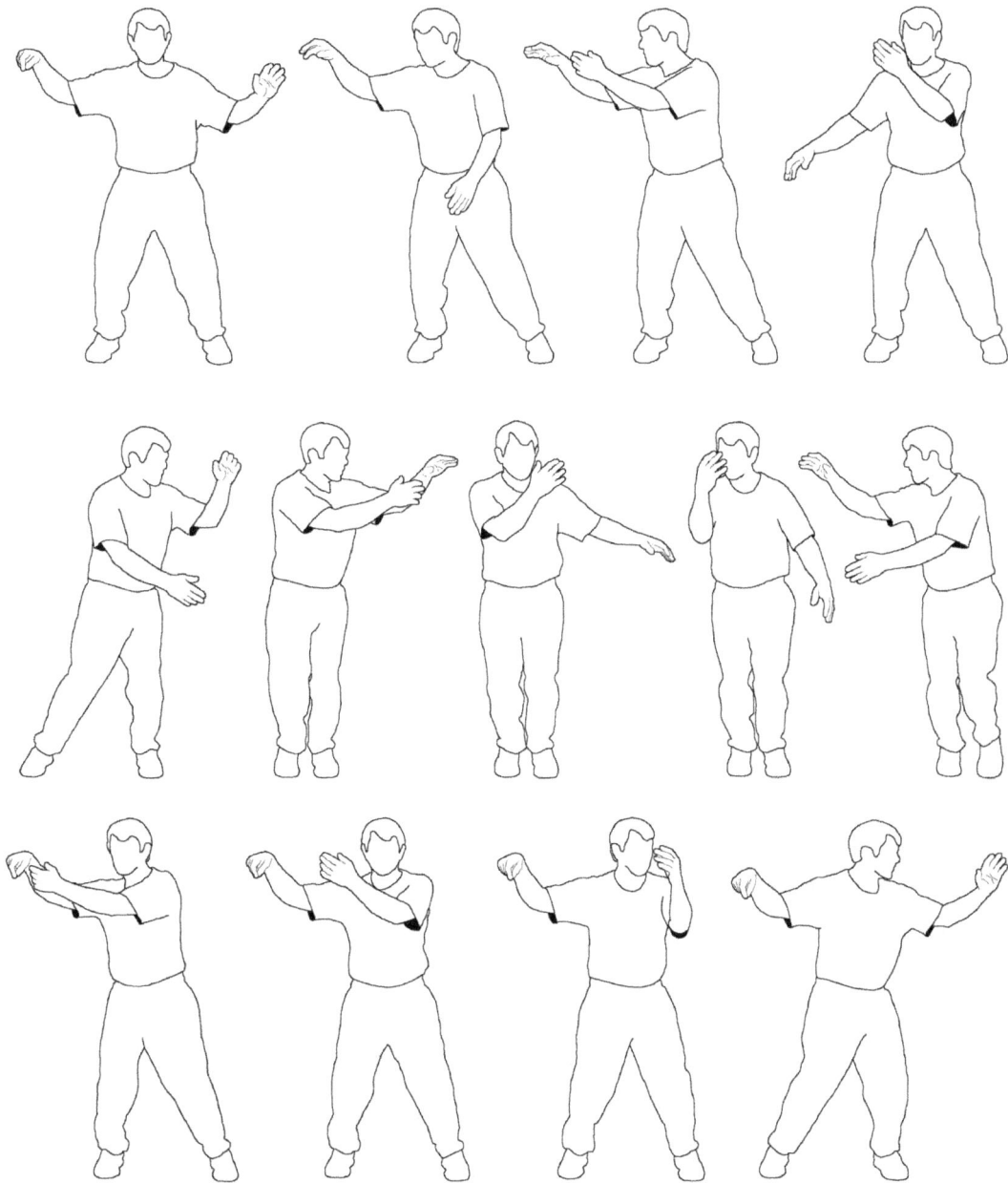

Figure 2.34 Both Wave Hands Like Clouds (top two rows) and Single Whip (bottom row) utilize Roll Back around all three vertical axes: central, right, and left.

# Press

**If Roll Back** was the simplest to comprehend, Press was, in many ways, the most difficult. Press is usually described as a compression energy, usually between the hands, that can be used to bounce away incoming energy, much as a drum head bounces off a coin tossed onto it. (Figure 2.35) I think it's often considered a compression of energy because when you do Press movements, it makes you feels as if you are both compressing your abdomen and squeezing something in the space between your arms or hands. But again, the usual description seemed to me to be defining a technique, not an energy, per se. Also, the yin aspect was absent. Armed with the idea that if the other three principal energies were in fact spherical/circular energies, then Press energy also must be spherical/circular.

After playing with Press for some time and analyzing where the energy was coming from and the way in which it moved, I realized that the clue to Press energy lies in the fact that in the classical Press posture, it is not the horizontal arm that generates the force but the arm that is pressing against, most often, the inside of the wrist of the horizontal arm. The key is that, unlike Ward Off, where the energy is generated in one leg

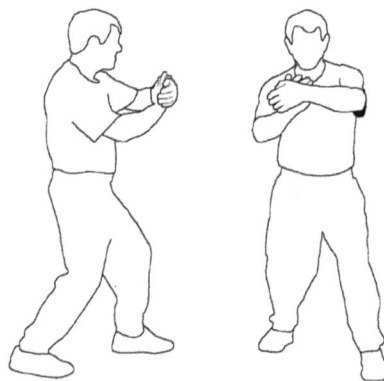

Figure 2.35 Press as a technique.

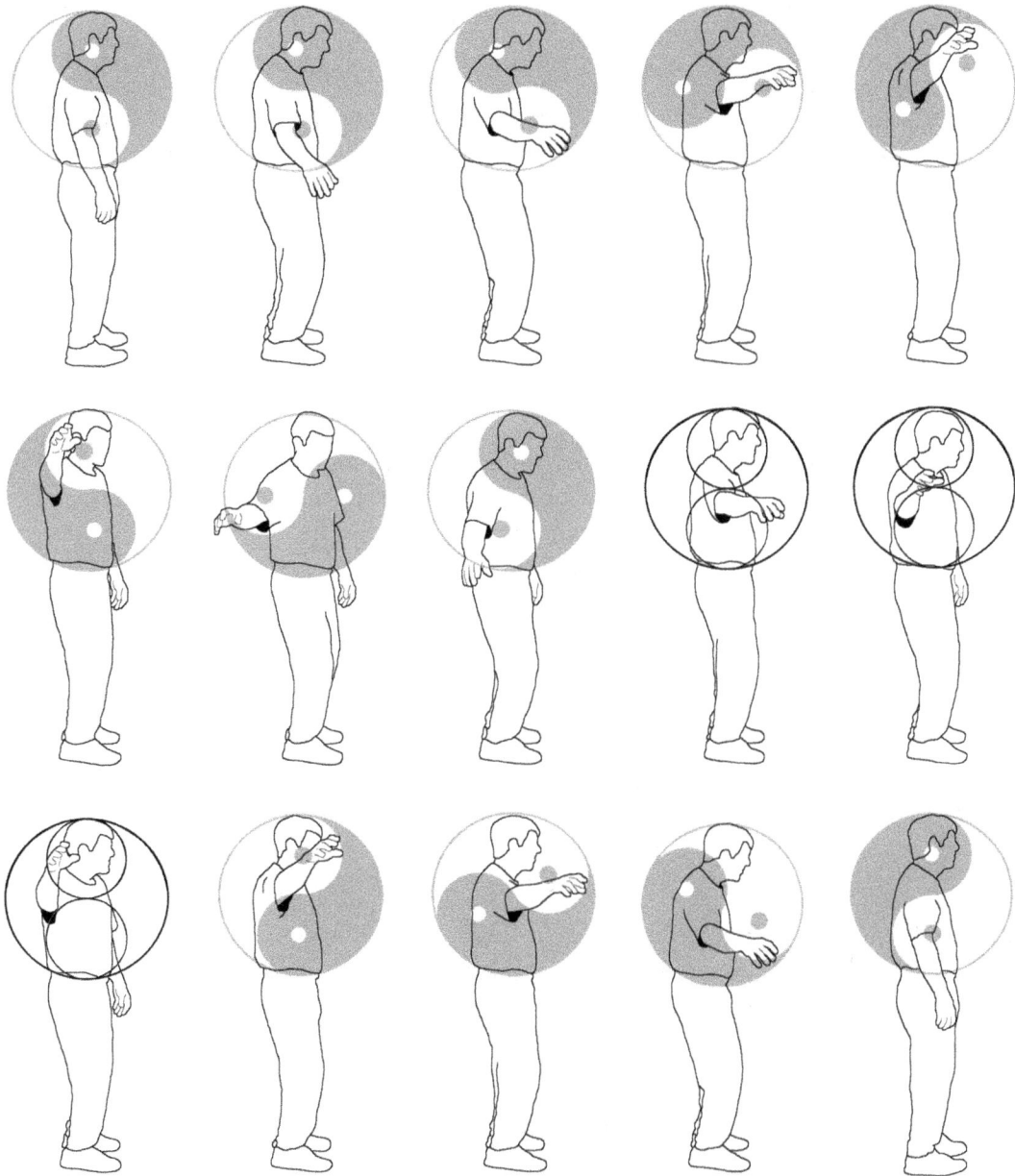

Figure 2.36 The Press circle rotates around one side or the other, in either direction. The spheres with the blank double fish indicate the moment when the energy switches direction.

and is expressed in the arm and hand of the opposite side, Press energy is generated by one leg and expressed in the arm and hand of the same side. When you get down to it, Press is generated by and occurs along and through one or the other of the side vertical axes. This makes the pure Press circle simply a large circle defined by the swing of the arm around the shoulder, either forward or backward, and

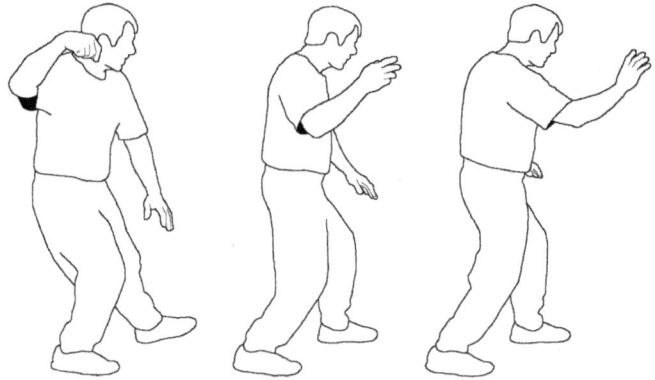

Figure 2.37 Brush Knee Twist Step is a common movement that utilizes Press energy, which begins in one leg and is delivered into the same-side arm.

that rotates on a plane that runs through either of the side vertical axes. (Figure 2.36)

Of course, this circling can't be accomplished through arm movement alone. That wouldn't be Tai Chi. The energetic center of the circle isn't the shoulder but the hip. The leg, moving up and down like a piston, drives the hip, which directs

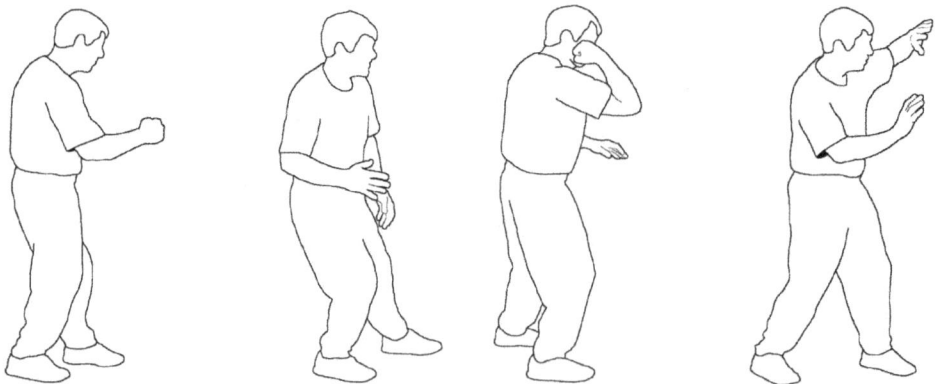

Figure 2.38 Press energy is evident in punches (left), many Elbow Strikes (center two), and even the twisty Maiden Pushing Shuttle (right).

the force into a vertically oriented circular path, rolling either forward or backward. The vertical rotation of the hip, in turn, propels the energy up through the same side of the torso, into the shoulder and, in some manner, into the arm to power a shove, strike, or other application.

This makes it obvious that Brush Knee Twist Step is a use of Press energy. (Figure 2.37) And so are Punch, most variants of Elbow Strike, and interestingly enough, Maiden Pushing Shuttle, which would be a fairly twisty version. (Figure 2.38) Press also can be used in an almost purely yin way to divert incoming energy by, say, swinging the arm in a backward circle to redirect a punch, which is fundamentally different than using Roll Back. (Figure 2.39)

However, the operation of Press is more complex than simply rotating force and energy through one side axis or the other. For Tai Chi movements to gain full power, they must engage the waist, which, among other things, helps to appropriately direct the power of the lower body into the upper body. In the other two vertically oriented Cardinal Energies—Push and Ward Off—the energy rising from the leg and into the torso naturally moves through the waist and Central Equilibrium—straight through it for Push and diagonally through it for Ward Off. But because Press is oriented around one side or the other, the energy coming up from the leg, through the torso, and into the arm doesn't directly engage Central Equilibrium or the waist, only the single side axis.

Press makes up for its lack of direct engagement with the waist in an ingenious

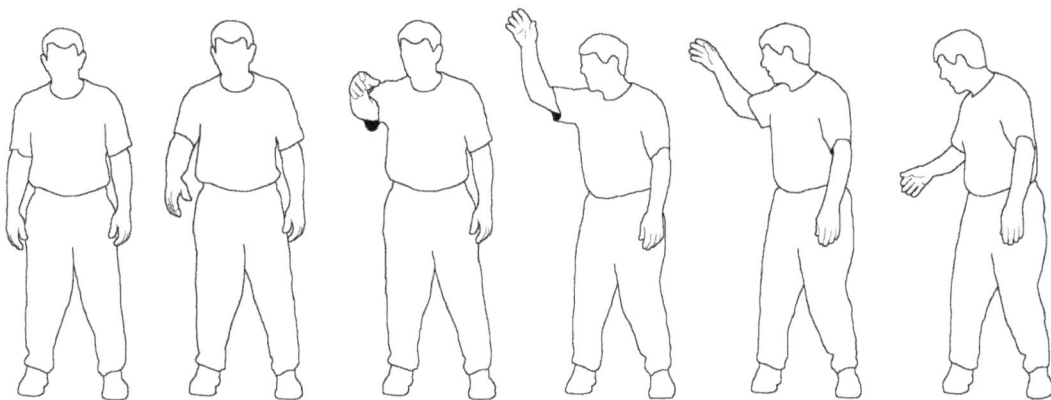

Figure 2.39 Using a backward swing of the arm to divert incoming energy is a yin aspect of Press.

fashion. The secret to this is in the yin arm—the horizontal arm in the classical Press posture, the "blocking" arm in Punch, Brush Knee Twist Step, and Maiden Pushing Shuttle, and the empty arm in an Elbow Strike. In each case, the yin arm moves perpendicularly, one way or the other, to the arm that is delivering the energy, depending on the particular Press variation. To Press forward, move the yin arm away from the yang arm, and to Press backwards, move the yin arm toward the yang arm. This isn't a case of the two arms moving independently of one another or in a stiff, angular way, but rather as if they are a single unit flexibly connected through the rotational point of one of the side vertical axes. When the yin arm begins to move, its flexible connection to the yang arm causes the yang arm

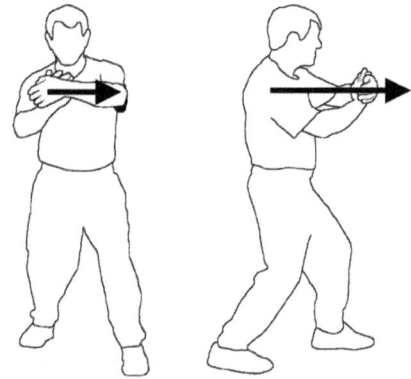

Figures 2.40 The classical Press posture showing force. The horizontal forearm pulls or jolts toward the elbow, propelling the back arm straight forward.

to move. And if you initiate the action by moving the yin arm first, instead of the yang arm, you enhance the whipping motion, either forward or backward.

Sometimes, the perpendicular movement of the yin arm is straight along the axis

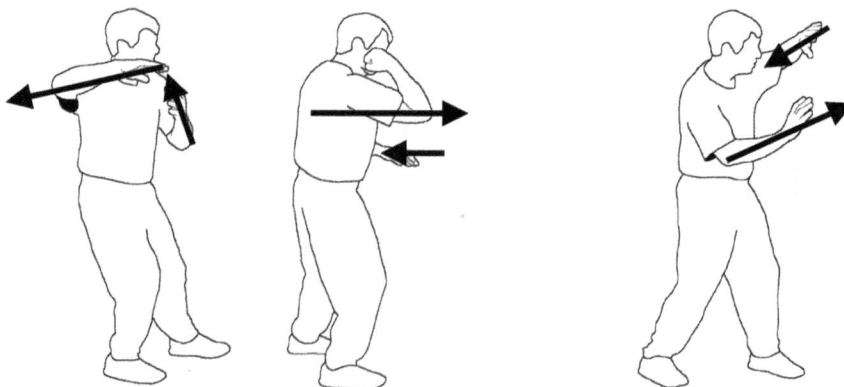

Figure 2.41 Two versions of Elbow Strike (left) and Maiden Pushing Shuttle (right) showing directions of leverage movement pivoting around the right vertical axis.

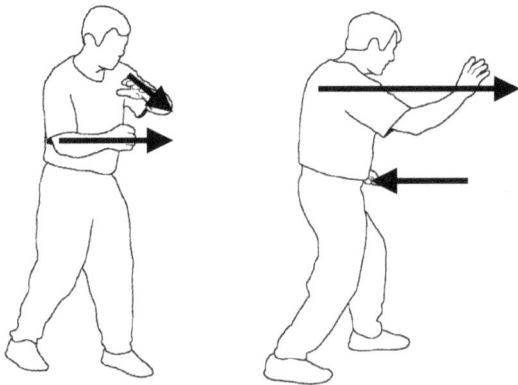

Figure 2.42 Punch and Brush Knee showing direction of leverage movement pivoting around the right vertical axis.

of its forearm. In the classical Press posture, for example, the horizontal forearm jerks along its axis from the hand toward the elbow, jolting the striking palm of the other hand forward. (Figure 2.40) The same basic dynamic occurs with Elbow Strike, whether forward or backward, and with Maiden Pushing Shuttle. (Figure 2.41) Sometimes the perpendicular movement entails swinging the yin arm away from the yang arm, as with Punch, where the swing tends to be small but tight, and Brush Knee Twist Step, where the swing tends to be larger. (Figure 2.42)

No matter which direction the motion of the yin hand goes or how compact its pull/push/swing, the dynamic is the same in that the nonstriking arm moves in a direction roughly perpendicular to the movement of the striking arm. And because of the flexible connection of the arms through the pivot point, this causes the body to rapidly rotate around the axis on the opposite side of the pushing/pulling arm, which in turn causes the yang arm on the same side as the axis to swiftly move forward or backward. (Figure 2.43) This is simply a matter of leverage, where a relatively mild force applied to the long arm of a lever produces a considerably larger effect on

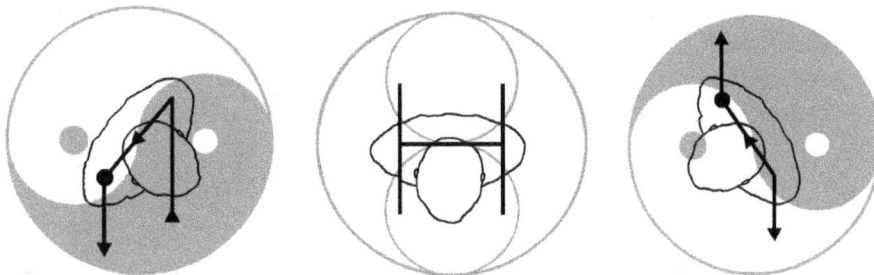

Figure 2.43 Press incorporates leverage around a side vertical axis. Press forward (left), neutral position (center), and Press backward (right). The dot indicates the pivot point.

the short arm of the lever. In the case of Press, the pivot point of the side vertical axis is the fulcrum, the yin arm is the long arm of the lever, and the yang arm is the short arm. Because the pulling/pushing/swinging arm generally performs its action over a longer distance due to the orientation of the body weight being swung on the opposite side from the pivot point, the subsequent thrust of the yang hand can be quite powerful even if its range is short. These movements must rotate around one of the side vertical axes to prevent double-weighting, which would occur if one tried to swing these movements around the central axis, which would force one to try to push from both feet simultaneously, eliminating both the waist movement and the leverage power and creating a condition of double-weighting.

All of the movements discussed above might be considered yang applications of Press energy, both forward and backward but the principle also holds true for yin applications such as wedding Press to Roll Back to pull or jerk someone inward or to the side and backward. Remember, any time you deliver forward energy, there is an equivalent backward energy involved that can be tapped. In all cases, whether forward or backward, the more severe the pull/push/swing of the yin arm, the sharper the jolt, strike, or pull of the yang arm.

> Only with vital essence, Qi and spirit intact, can one peacefully ponder the intellectual and be prepared to mobilize the martial. Through quietude and mobilization, one can develop and transform through the intellectual and martial to achieve spiritual wisdom. Those of the past who achieved perception could transcend material phenomena through these teachings.... When the self-cultivation reaches the head, then the person will be successful in both martial and intellectual aspects.
>
> —Wu Kung Cho[8]

# Conclusion

**In short, the** four Cardinal Energies, in their purest forms, are simply using the legs to push the body in certain directions, using that impetus to rotate the hips and waist, then using that rotation to swing the arms through all the basic circles they can make.

> Push = rotating straight forward or backward from the central vertical axis
> Roll Back = rotating side to side around one of the three vertical axes
> Ward Off = rotating from the leg of either side, diagonally across the body, and into the arm on the opposite side, often from the vertical axis of one side, through the central axis, to the axis of the opposite side
> Press = rotating from the leg of one side into the arm on the same side, always through the vertical axis of either the right or the left side (Figure 2.44)

Each Cardinal Energy, in its pure form, is a sphere, but once the sphere is given rotation, the most powerful expression of each is along a circular plane around the sphere's outmost circumference—its equator—in the direction of rotation. Furthermore, each sphere/circle can rotate forward to expel energy or backward to draw in energy. However, there are instances, depending on one's intention, where the backward rotation delivers energy, as in Elbow Strike, and the forward rotation draws in the opponent, as when using Brush Knee Twist Step as a throw.

Press (through side axis)
or
Push (through central axis)

Ward Off

Press

Push

Ward Off

Roll Back

Roll Back

Ward Off

Roll Back

Push

Press

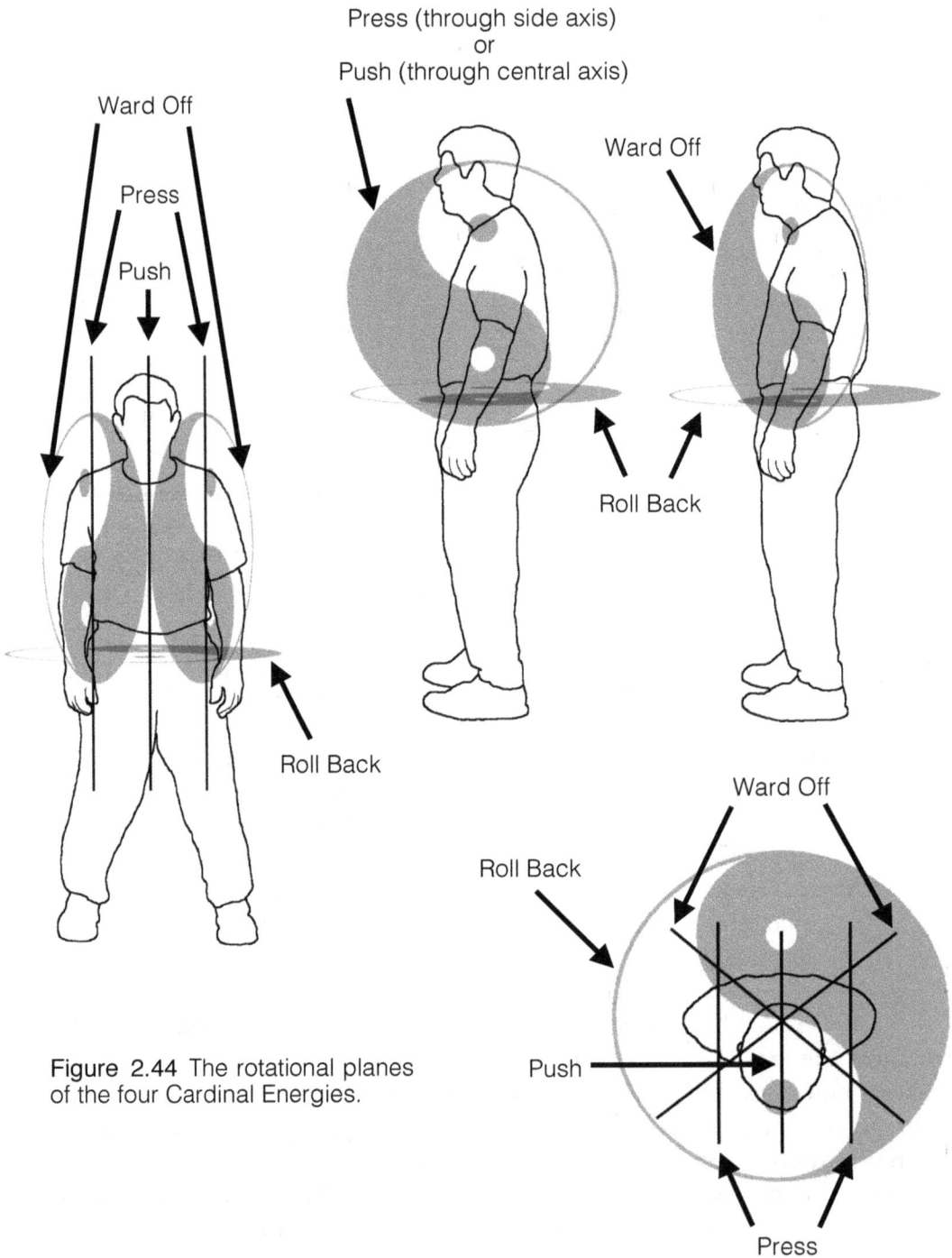

Figure 2.44 The rotational planes
of the four Cardinal Energies.

And of course, the circles of the four Cardinal Energies don't operate independently of the body. Sure, you can swing your arms around these circles without engaging much of the body beyond the shoulders, but this would not be Tai Chi. In fact, as the Tai Chi Classics tell us, any movement of the upper body is initiated by the legs and transferred by the hips and waist to the upper body, which then responds. I'll cover this in greater depth in the chapter on Chan-ssu Chin.

These spheres/circles are the Cardinal Energies in their purest forms, but they are rarely expressed in their purest forms in the Tai Chi movements or in applications of the movements against an opponent. For that, we'll have to look at the way the circles are altered to make them martially effective—and to assume characteristics of the tai chi symbol from which the art derives its name. The way into that discussion is an examination of the four Ordinal Energies.

> Tai Chi Ch'uan, according to popular beliefs, is undoubtedly the supreme achievement of Chang San-Feng, who, at the end of the Sung Dynasty, revolutionized and synthesized all the systems in existence and created the so-called "Exoteric system." What makes it unique as it is practiced now is its systemic training of the mind (spirit) as well as the body.
>
> —Wen-shan Huang[9]

# The Ordinal Energies

**The four Ordinal** Energies—Shoulder Strike, Elbow Strike, Pull/Pluck, and Split—are generally described as techniques that tap into or combine the four Cardinal Energies. (Figure 2.45) We saw in the previous section, for example, how Elbow Strike often combines Press with Roll Back. But the Ordinal Energies aren't just a primer on the ways that the Cardinal Energies can be used in combination, for there is an aspect to them that makes them crucial enough to consider them equal in importance to the Cardinal Energies. In a sense, the idea behind this also ought to contradict the association of the Ordinal Energies with the four corners of the square.

When we look at the Cardinal Energies, we see that three of them—Push, Ward Off, and Press—are primarily vertically oriented, while one—Roll Back—is horizontally oriented. As we've discovered, the vertically oriented Cardinal Energies roll one's sphere of energy in various ways both forward and backward along planes that actually cover the ordinal directions as well as the cardinal ones: Ward Off goes corner to corner; Push goes straight forward and backward, also implying straight side-to-side; and Press delineates the side walls of the bounding square within which Ward Off and Push operate. It is Roll Back that truly defines the Ordinal Energies because it embodies the circling of the square, and through its horizontal rotation, it can engage with all three of the vertical energies.

Before we can go further, though, we need to discuss a couple of interlinked concepts, and we'll start with Tai Chi's prohibition against double-weighting. The Tai Chi Classics frequently mention double-weighting as a major fault and enjoin the practitioner to avoid it. But what is double-weighting, exactly? The Tai Chi Classics put it like this: "The weight of the body should rest on just one foot. If the

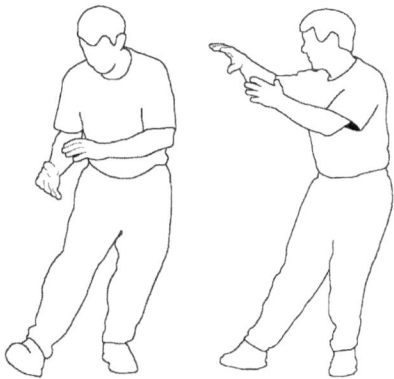

**Pull / Pluck**
(Cai, wind, northwest)
A pulling energy, low and high

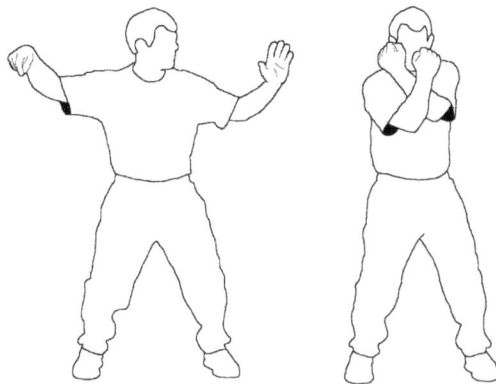

**Split**
(Lie, thunder, southeast)
An energy that moves apart from the center
or toward the center from the sides.

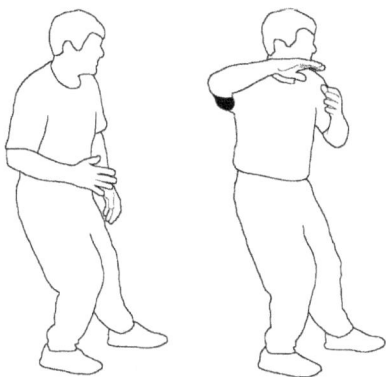

**Elbow Strike**
(Zhou, lake, northeast)
Elbow striking energy,
low and high

**Shoulder Strike**
(Kao, mountain, southwest)
Full-body striking energy with the
shoulder or any other part of the torso

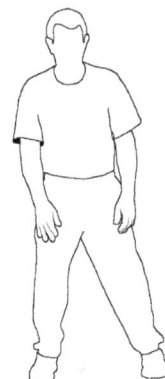

Figure 2.45 The Four Ordinal Energies (ordinal directions).

weight is divided between the two feet, this is double-weightedness."[10] Thus, the basic explanation of double-weighting is that the weight of the Tai Chi practitioner should be primarily on either one leg or the other or should constantly shift from one leg to the other. Only rarely does the weight fall equally on both feet, for example in Open Tai Chi and the beginning of White Crane Preens Wing, and most of these instances are transitional and fleeting. It also is said that to properly issue or receive energy, the Tai Chi practitioner must launch his attack or retreat from a firm stance on one leg while emptying the other side. In addition, if you need to advance or retreat and you are double-weighted, you must first shift your weight to one leg or the other before you can step, which delays the advance or evasion. This process is automatically taken care of in a single-weighted stance, making advance and retreat quicker because they don't involve shifting the weight first. These are all excellent reasons to avoid double-weighting in its simplest incarnation.

But while it is important that the practitioner's weight constantly shift back and forth from one leg to the other or that an attack or defense be accomplished from a single-weighted stance, these are only the most basic reasons to avoid double-weighting. To delve deeper, we have to look at how Tai Chi produces force. In Tai Chi, an attack or counter is composed of two elements of force: linear force and torque. Linear force is born out of the flattened circles of the three vertical Cardinal Energies—Ward Off, Press, and Push. I'm calling this force linear not because it travels in a dead-straight line, which wouldn't look much like Tai Chi, but because it is created and manifests along a single plane defined by the Tai Chi sphere's rotating equator or as tangents thrown from the circles those spheres create. This linear force is produced by the pushing of the yang leg and the vertical circling of the yang hip. It then is directed by the waist through the torso and into the appropriate arm, as noted in the prior descriptions of the three vertical Cardinal Energies.

Torque, which is imparted by adding Roll Back to develop the coiling and twisting of the Ordinal Energies, "is the tendency of a force to rotate an object around an axis. Just as a force is a push or a pull [linear force], torque can be thought of as a twist to an object."[11] Torque can manifest in two ways—as usual, the yin and yang of things. First, it can be created by applying a linear force at right angles to an axis of rotation to create spin or twist. A good example can be seen in the turning force of a wrench tightening a nut onto a bolt. Second, an axis that spins up from a still state also produces torque that manifests outwardly. This can be seen in the twisting effect produced by an engine or motor that is either just turned on or whose speed is suddenly revved up.

Direction of Rotation

Direction of Force

Neutral

Yang

Neutral

Yin

Neutral

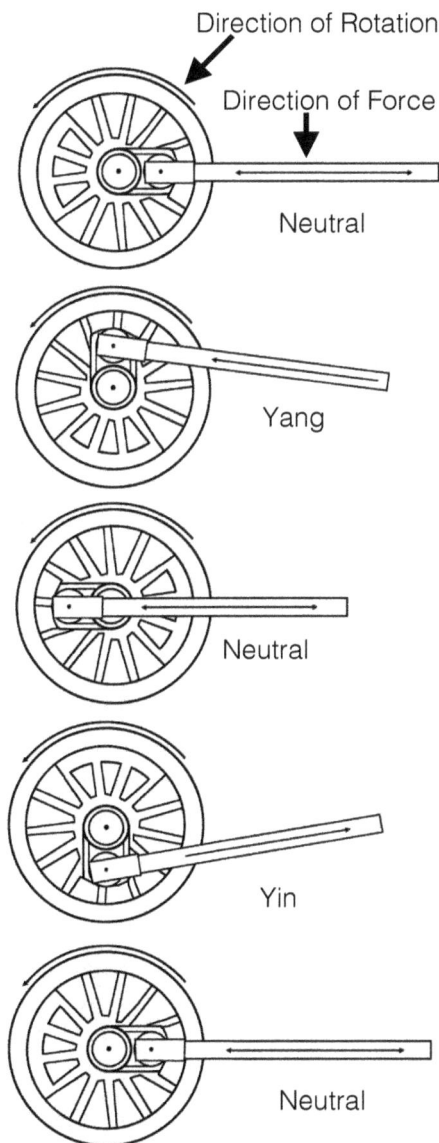

Figure 2.46 The driving wheel of a locomotive illustrates the way the body converts linear force into circular movement and vice versa. (Forces are from the perspective of the piston driving the wheel, and they would be reversed if the wheel were driving the piston.)

Both of these aspects are present in the driving wheel of a locomotive, which, like Tai Chi, uses an offset of linear force in relation to an axis of rotation. (Figure 2.46) Normally, the wheel is spun using the linear force of the thrusting and counter-thrusting piston to create spin. But it also is possible to spin the wheel to drive the piston back and forth.

In Tai Chi, torque is extremely important. Up to this point, I've been describing the movement of the Cardinal Energies as linear because these energies, in their pure forms, produce cycles and tangents along discreet planes: Push, straight forward/backward from the middle; Press, forward/backward on one side or the other; Ward Off, diagonally forward/backward from one side to the other; and Roll Back to the right/left on the horizontal plane. (See Figure 2.44 on page 68.) However, we've also seen that movement along these planes is circular, and circular movement must spin or rotate around an axis: Push, Press, and Ward Off around an axis that runs horizontally through the hips and Roll Back around one or more of the vertical axes (central, right, or left).

The difference in the axes of rotation of the three vertically oriented Cardinal Energies and the horizontally oriented Roll Back allows Roll Back to operate—and cooperate—with each of the vertical planes, but there are restrictions. Both Ward Off, whose diagonal spin goes from one side to the other, and Press, whose rotation is offset to the side, can utilize torque from Roll Back because the axes of their rotations do not conflict with the axis of Roll Back's rotation. But Roll Back can't actually operate with Push because Push is an energy whose plane rotates straight forward and backward from Central Equilibrium, and Roll Back rotates around Central Equilibrium. The two rotations, being at right angles to each other through and around the same axis, can't occur simultaneously. Similarly, the three vertical planes all use the same axis of rotation and thus cannot operate simultaneously with each other—you can't Press and Ward Off at the same time, for example. But even so, all three vertical energies can be linked sequentially through Roll Back to allow them to cooperate together or in sequence without conflict.

It is useful here, to visualize a locomotive's driving wheel replacing the rotating tai chi symbols depicted in the previous sections on the Eight Gates. In the cases of Push, Press, and Ward Off, the driving wheel is oriented vertically along each of these planes, and in the case of Roll Back, the driving wheel lies on the horizontal plane. This makes it obvious that Push, Press, and Ward Off create linear force by rotating forward and backward along their vertical planes, and Roll Back creates torquing force, forward or backward, by twisting the body on the horizontal plane, around a vertical axis. The torquing also involves lowering one's body weight onto the yang leg—an action often called "sitting," "sinking," or "settling"—then driving the leg upward. This propels the energy through the forward or backward circling of the hip, through the waist, into the torso, and from there, into the appropriate arm in the appropriate manner. The horizontal torquing is actuated by a twist of the waist around a vertical axis—usually around the hip of the weight-bearing leg, which pushes the hip against the base of the torso as the torso turns around it.

This can happen only with rotation around one of the vertical axes, so we can see again why Roll Back can't operate directly with Push, which has no transverse rotation. This also makes it clear how important it is to avoid double-weighting, for the fault of pushing with both legs in Ward Off or Press movements would prevent the waist from rotating on the horizontal plane, effectively disabling Roll Back's torquing function.

The key here is that the body can execute movement around the horizontal axis that connects the two hips and one, or a sequence, of the three vertical axes. This is because the joints and connections of the hips and spine act like a complex universal joint and differential gear. Now, visualize two locomotive driving wheels oriented at right angles to one another and sharing a common piston. The vertical wheel

—Press or Ward Off—provides spin along an upright plane, and the horizontal wheel—Roll Back—provides torque along a flat plane. Together, they drive their common piston forward or backward, and the combined forces are far greater in power than either is alone, and certainly a quantum leap in power over simple, straightforward linear acceleration. All Ward Off and Press movements employ both vertical circling and horizontal torque, though they might not be expressed equally. Using Monkey Moving Backward as a strike or tripping shove emphasizes the vertical aspect, while using it as a throw emphasizes the horizontal aspect. (Figure 2.47) Push movements only employ vertical spin, but they compensate for the lack of horizontal torque by being able to utilize the power of the leg muscles and the entire body weight expressed straight along the centerline.

From the above, we can see that the Ordinal Energies are actually composed of circling along one of the three vertical planes in combination with torquing around the horizontal plane, each of which feeds its energy into a combined focal point. But even though spin is a circular force, its expression along the vertical planes tends to produce linear results because of the forward/backward orientation of movement along those planes. It is Roll Back—the circling of the square—that gives Tai Chi its transverse torquing capabilities. So it seems to me that maybe the the Cardinal Energies ought to be called the Directional Energies, and the Ordinal Energies ought to be called the Circular Energies, for it is within them that torque is emphasized. For the sake of clarity and tradition, however, I'm not going to rock the boat and will stick with the names Cardinal and Ordinal Energies.

Martially, training the legs, body core, and arms to simultaneously or sequentially circle and torque inward or outward is what gives Tai Chi its characteristic coiling, uncoiling, and cork-screwing movements that allow the practitioner to gather and release large amounts of force and power within compressed spaces. The Ordinal Energies also provide ways to divert an opponent's incoming energy away from oneself or to spiral that energy, and more, back into the opponent. The power of the Ordinal Energies is usually quite sharp and jolting and can easily and severely injure an opponent or training partner.

Now, let's look at each of the Ordinal Energies, beginning with the simplest: Shoulder Strike.

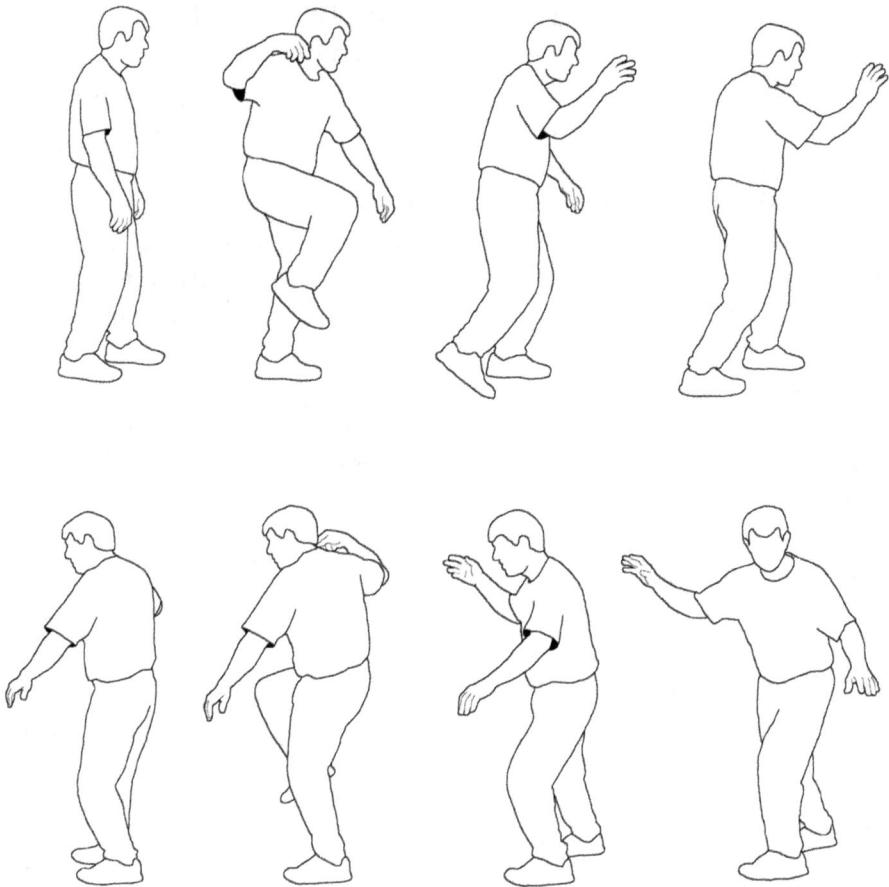

**Figure 2.47** When used as a strike or shove, Monkey Moving Backward emphasizes vertical spin (top row), but when it is used as a throw, it emphasizes horizontal torque (second row).

# Shoulder Strike

**Although Shoulder Strike** is, in some of its aspects, one of the more difficult of the Ordinal Energies to perform accurately, it is the easiest to understand because at its base, it is simply pushing off one or the other foot and slamming some part of your torso into your opponent. (Figure 2.48)

The slam is focused and controlled so that the force coming from the foot and leg is delivered with the entire body and you do not go off balance when you do the slamming. The slam can be hard, jolting, and penetrating, or it can be softer, more elastic, and repelling. Most commonly, the shoulder is used, but the slam could be with the back, hip, or side, all of which require more refined control than using the shoulder, which is pretty easy. In all cases, the linear force surging up the leg is directed by the waist to the appropriate strike point—even when it is the hip, which lies below the waist, that is doing the strike, the movement is directed by the waist.

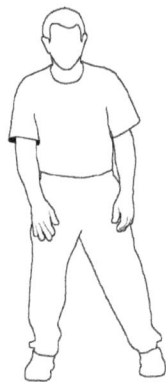

In the form I do, Shoulder Strike is implied in Grasping Bird's Tail and several other movements and is expressed overtly in several Shoulder Strike movements within the form. It works well with Ward Off (using the opposite shoulder) and Push

Figure 2.48 In Shoulder Strike, the energy that begins in one leg is expressed in some part of the torso—here, from the left leg into the right shoulder.

(using the upper back) and only weakly with Press (using the same-side shoulder). Roll Back, of course, is what rotates the body, however slightly, to impart torque to the strike when using either Ward Off or Press to perform the strike, but as noted earlier, Roll Back can't function in direct conjunction with Push since the two forces are expressed at perpendicular angles to one another. Push must rely on the weight of the body to compensate for its lack of transverse torque.

The "four techniques," above and below, divide into Heaven and earth.
Pull-down, Split, Elbow-stroke and Shoulder-stroke each have their origin and object.
Pull-down being Heaven and Shoulder-stroke earth, they mutually respond to each other.
Why should we care if above and below do not complement each other?
If Split and Elbow-stroke are practiced too far apart,
One will lose the relation of Ch'ien [Heaven], and K'un [earth] and will lament it forever.
This theory explains the planes of Heaven and earth.
When advancing use Elbow-stroke and Split, with the arms in the shape of the character for man [i.e., bent].

—Wang Tsung-yueh[12]

# Elbow Strike

**Elbow Strike also** is fairly easy to understand in its basic form. The elbow can strike backward anywhere between shoulder height and hip height. It also can strike forward, upward, sideways—any way, in fact, that you can swing and strike with the elbow. (Figure 2.49) Actually, Elbow Strike can be extended to any blow or block delivered with the elbow or forearm.

We discussed the use of Press energy in combination with Roll Back to power Elbow Strike in the section on Press, and this probably is the most common combina-

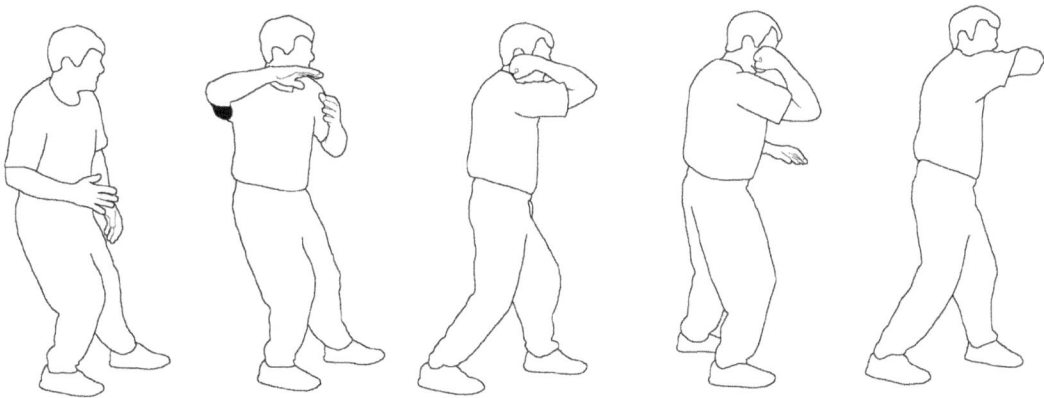

Figure 2.49 Elbow Strike can be done at any level between shoulder and hip, either forward, backward, or to either side.

tion. But Elbow Strike also works well with Ward Off. This can be seen in the movement Beating Tiger, where you can swing your body weight down and up to use the forearm to block upward or to slam the forearm into an opponent's chest or chin. (Figure 2.50) Another example of Elbow Strike being used as a block is Seven Stars from the form I do, where the vertical forearm swings sideways against the arm of an incoming punch to divert it. (Figure 2.51) However, this same movement also can be used to deliver a chop or whipping hammer fist. More complexly, the elbow or forearm can be used as a fulcrum for joint locks, throws, and back fist strikes.

Because Elbow Strike uses Roll Back to twist around one or more of the vertical axes to develop torque, it does not work well with Push, which simply rolls the Tai Chi sphere forward or backward and does not rotate it either direction sideways to develop torque.

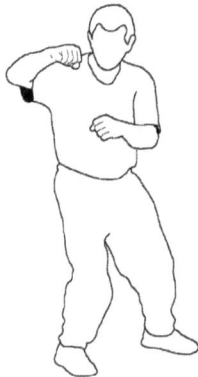

Figure 2.50 Beating Tiger is a complex movement that can use Elbow Strike in a couple of ways: as an upward block to open the way for a lower-hand punch, or to strike laterally with the forearm.

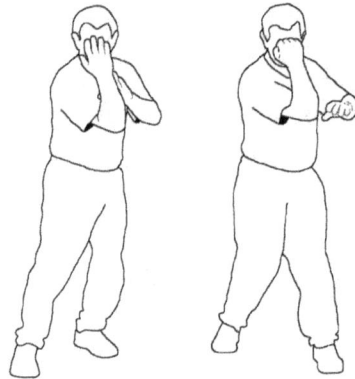

Figure 2.51 Seven Stars can use the elbow/forearm to divert an incoming punch to one side or to deliver a chop or hammer fist.

# Pull / Pluck

**Pull/Pluck requires** a bit of explanation because it functions in a couple of fairly different ways. Most people just call it Pull or Pluck, but you'll see in a moment why I include both terms. At its basic, Pull/Pluck is used to pull or twist your opponent off balance in some way, such as down and forward or to the side. (Figure 2.52) This is the Pull aspect. The Pluck aspect can be used to grasp and hold or pull some body part in some direction—an incoming arm, for example. (Figure 2.53) Usually, the pulling or plucking is done with the hand, but it doesn't have to be. It can be a trapping with the crook of a joint, most commonly the wrist, but sometimes the crook of the elbow, the armpit, and even the crook of the knee.

Pull and Pluck can be differentiated in the same way that a baseball player orients his glove to catch an incoming ball. If the ball arrives above the player's waist, the player points the fingers of his glove upward, and if it arrives below his waist, he points his fingers downward. Similarly, the Pull function

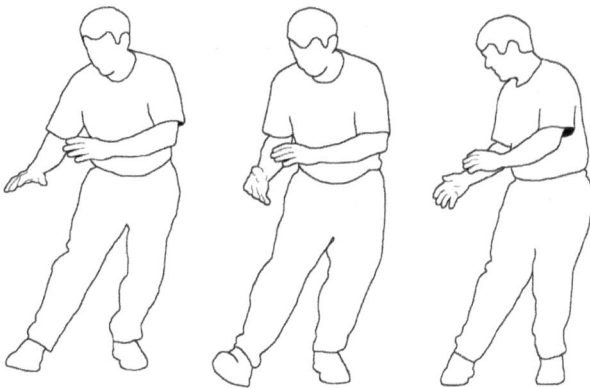

**Figure 2.52** Pull is used below the waist.

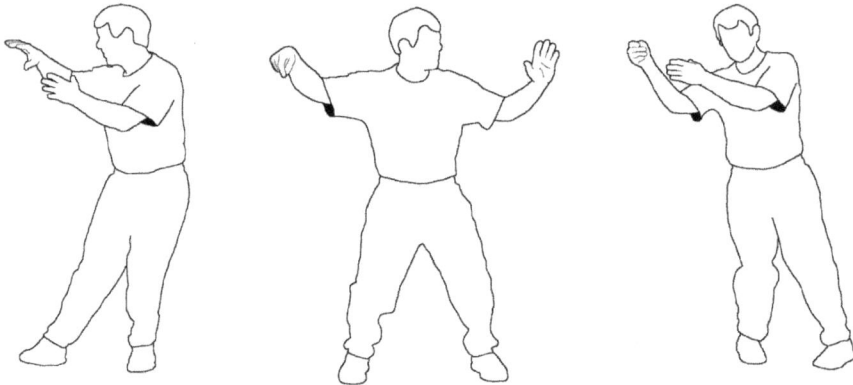

Figure 2.53 Pluck is used above the waist.

generally is performed when dealing with energy below the waist: pulling incoming energy inward and downward or to the side. The Pluck function happens when dealing with energy approaching above the waist: plucking the incoming energy to one side or the other, sometime along an upward or downward trajectory.

In addition, in Pluck, the grasp is done with the thumb, forefinger, and middle finger. It is similar to the closing of pincers. Pull, on the other hand, uses the middle, ring, and pinky fingers to do the grasping. This is interesting in that the thumb, forefinger, and half of the middle finger are activated by the nerves (primarily the median nerve) that run from shoulder to fingers along the inside of the arm, while the pinky, ring, and other half of the middle finger are activated by the nerves (primarily the ulnar nerve) that run from the fingers to shoulder along the outside of the arm. You can feel this in your own body in a practical way. If you grasp your wrist with the thumb and first two fingers of your other hand and pull, you can feel the pull coming from the top front side of your shoulder, and if you pull with the last three fingers, you can feel the pull coming from the bottom back side of the shoulder. So essentially, when you Pluck, you do so from the top outside of the shoulder, and when you Pull, you do so from the bottom inside of the shoulder.

Dynamically, the areas where the energy comes from in Pull versus Pluck helps define how you utilize your body when doing each. Pluck primarily rotates Roll Back, combined with either Ward Off or Press, straight back on one side or the other. Pull demonstrates a sinking or sitting motion that combines Roll Back with

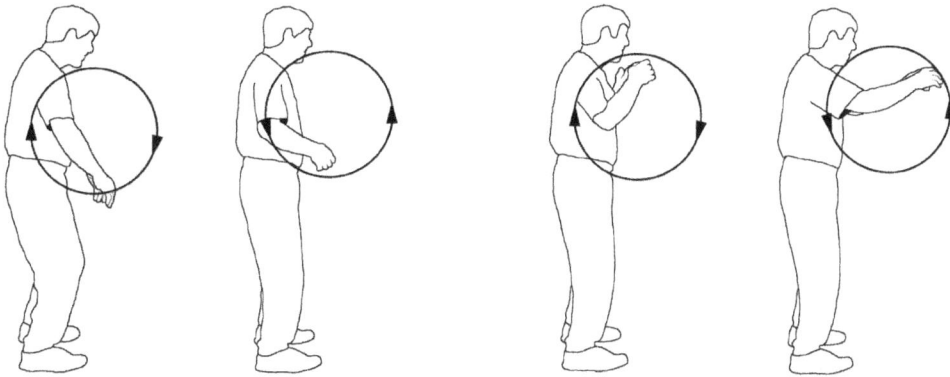

Figure 2.54 Pull and Pluck work co-operatively together, either forward or backward, around the Push circle.

Ward Off or Press along a downward-slanting trajectory. And both Pull and Pluck can be used with Push in a few instances—usually circularly, down or up, right in front of you, substituting a sinking of the body weight for Roll Back.

Pull/Pluck is generally considered to be a yin energy because it draws the opponent into emptiness, but it, too, has a yang aspect. A Pull backward or to the side, for example, automatically includes a backward Elbow Strike, and the back of a Plucking wrist can be used to block an opponent's strike or to strike his face or head. Also, the fingertips of the plucking hand can be used to strike vulnerable areas.

Pull/Pluck works very well with Roll Back and Ward Off (Figures 2.52 & 2.53), and it also works in a few instances with Push, particularly along Push's downward curve, either forward or backward. (Figure 2.54) Another example that employs the Push circle is Needle Sinks to Sea Bottom, which can be used as either a Pull or a Pluck, depending on your purpose. (Figure 2.55) Pull/Pluck also works with Press in movements like Brush Knee Twist Step, where the nonstriking hand pulls down or redirects the opponent's striking hand (Figure 2.56), or in Punch, where the nonstriking hand can pull the opponent into the punch. (Figure 2.57) An unusual usage of Pull/Pluck is its combination with Press in the odd movement following Golden Cock that seems to be found only in Wu Family and Northern Wu styles. (Figure 2.58) This movement will be described in greater detail in the next section.

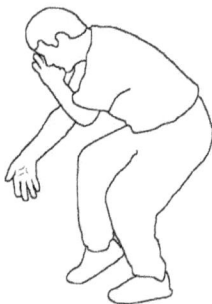

Figure 2.55 Needle Sinks to Sea Bottom is an example of Pull/Pluck that combines with the Push sphere rolled forward and down.

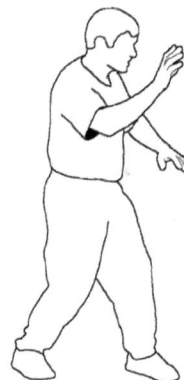

Figure 2.56 In the Press movement of Brush Knee Twist Step, the blocking hand can pull down an opponent's attacking arm.

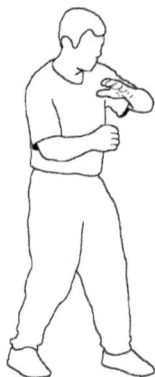

Figure 2.57 In the Press movement of Punch, the nonstriking hand pulls the opponent into the punch.

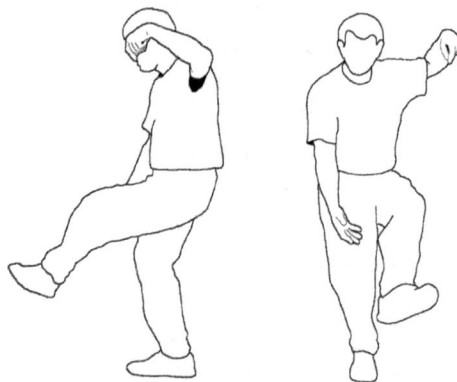

Figure 2.58 In this movement, which follows Golden Cock Stands on One Leg in Wu and Northern Wu styles, Pluck is combined with Press.

# Split

**Split is one** of the most complex and interesting of the Eight Gates. At its most obvious, Split happens when the energy starts in the middle and moves apart in opposite directions—sometimes equally, sometimes emphasizing one side or the other. A couple of examples found in most forms are Single Whip (Figure 2.59) and Slant Flying. (Figure 2.60) However, to add a yin dimension to these yang movements, the arms also can come together equally or nearly so. (Figure 2.61) This is evident in the posture of the form I do called Seven Stars (Figure 2.62), which is similar in form and function to the posture usually called Play Guitar or Ready Posture or in the more-common Twin Peeks Between the Ears.

Another good example is Monkey Moving Backward as performed in the form I

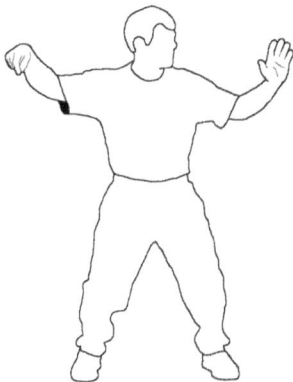

Figure 2.59 Single Whip is a Split that combines Roll Back with both Ward Off and Pull/Pluck.

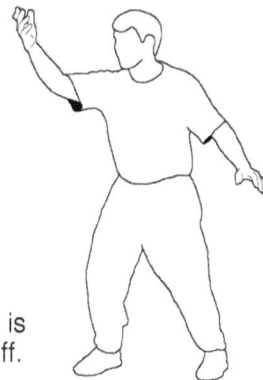

Figure 2.60 Slant Flying is a Split that uses Ward Off.

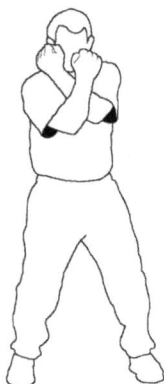

Figure 2.61 In the yin aspect of Split, the arms come together instead of separating.

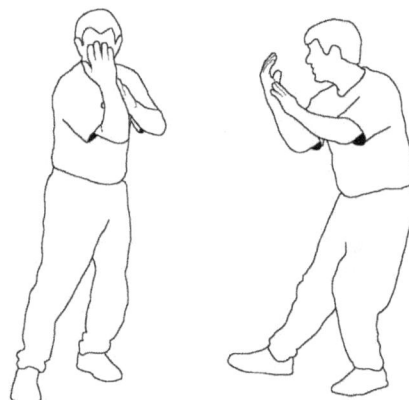

Figure 2.62 Seven Stars is an example of a yin Split.

do. Looking at terminal photos of Monkey Moving Backward and Brush Knee Twist Step, the two would seem to be indistinguishable, but the way each moves the energy in getting into this posture is very different. Brush Knee Twist Step clearly utilizes Press energy because the force begins in the rear foot, moves through the leg and torso of the same side, and ends in the hand of the same side. (Figure 2.63) In Monkey Moving Backward, however, the force begins in the waist and moves simultaneously into the rear leg and one or the other hand. If it is directed into the same-side hand, it uses Press, but if it is directed into the opposite side hand, it uses Ward Off. The former would generally be a yang application that can be used, say, as a strike or tripping shove. (Figure 2.64) The latter would generally be a yin application that can be used, say, as a backward-moving throw. (Figure 2.65)

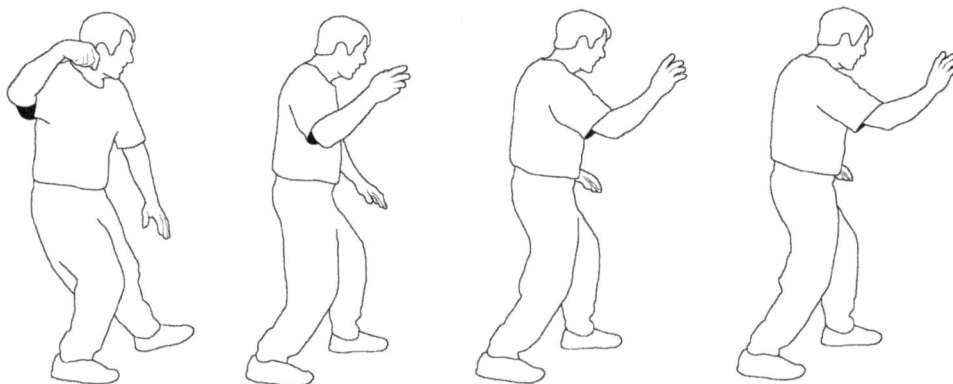

Figure 2.63 Brush Knee Twist Step is a Press movement because the energy begins in the foot of one leg then travels through the torso into the same-side arm.

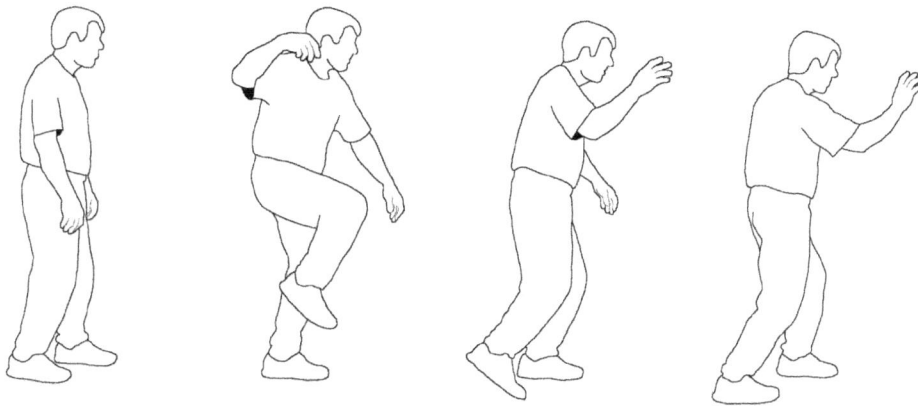

Figure 2.64 Monkey Moving Backward is a Split movement because the energy begins in the waist/hip and moves into both a leg and an arm simultaneously. Here is an example of yang Monkey Moving Backward using Press energy to execute a strike or a tripping shove, in which the energy travels through the leg and the same-side arm.

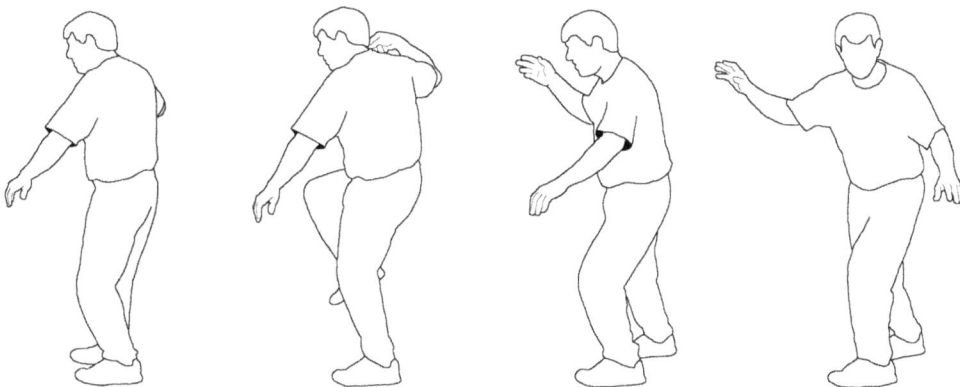

Figure 2.65 A yin Monkey Moving Backward using Ward Off energy can function as a backward throw. In this case, the energy begins in the waist/hip and moves into the same-side leg and the opposite-side arm.

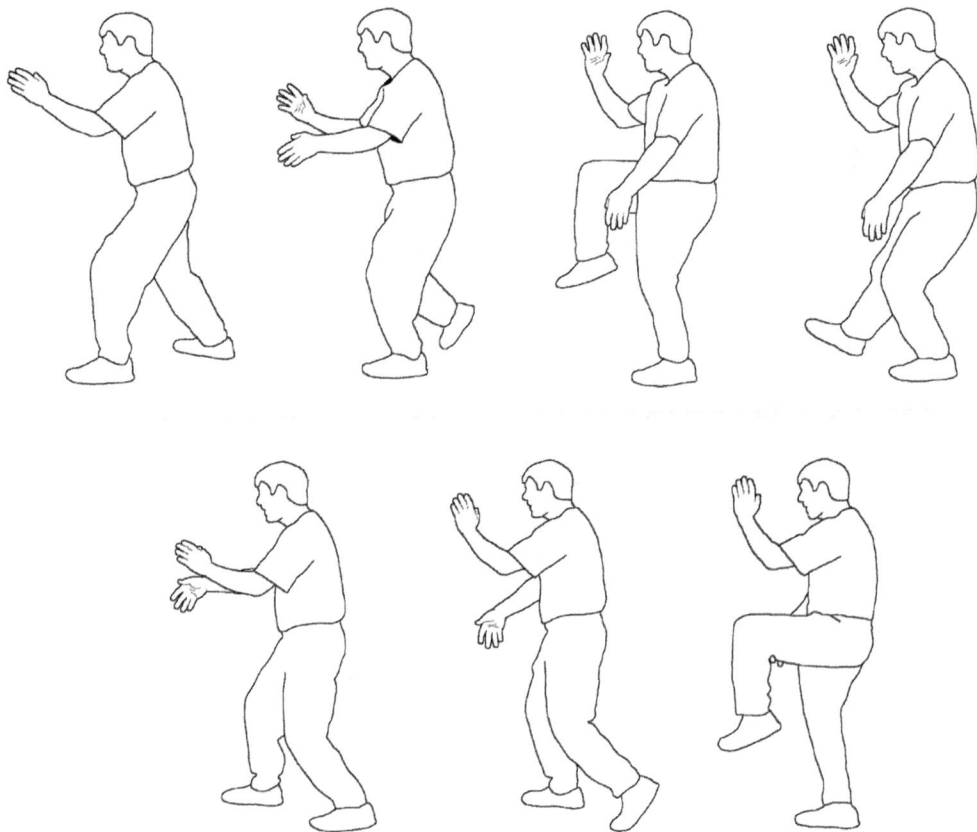

**Figure 2.66** Golden Cock Stands on One Leg is a rare example of Split being used with Push energy.

However, whether used in a yang or yin fashion, the energy of Split still begins in the middle and moves in two opposite directions at once or begins on two opposite sides and draws in toward the middle. In Monkey Moving Backward, it starts in the hip/waist area and moves simultaneously toward the pushing foot and one or the other hand. In Single Whip, it opens the arms in two directions around the central axis of the spine. In Twin Peaks Between the Ears, it closes the arms equally from two directions around the central axis.

Golden Cock Stands on One Leg is a rare instance of Split being used with Push. (Figure 2.66) As one comes out of Snake Creeps Down and rises onto the left leg, one raises the right knee and the right arm, while the left hand dives downward. The opposing separation of the two arms and the two legs is the Split aspect, and at first, it seems like it is being used in conjunction with Ward Off since the upward force appears to move from the left leg into the right hand. However, since Golden Cock is played directly in front of the body rather than on a diagonal, it taps into the straight-forward/straight-backward rotation that is indicative of Push. The movement is repeated by stepping forward onto the right leg and lifting the left side while sinking the right side, repeating the Split, again in conjunction with Push energy.

That is immediately followed by that odd movement that seems to occur only in Wu Family and Northern Wu styles that I mentioned in the previous section. (Figure 2.67) In this movement, one remains standing on the right leg and the energy moves simultaneously from the waist to the left foot, causing it to kick diagonally forward with the cocked-back sole, and through the left arm, creating a backward pulling/plucking motion with the left hand. I'll return to the strangeness of this movement later when I discuss the Tai Chi bow, but it is sufficient here to see that the force, although seemingly executed diagonally across the body, actually is generated and expressed along one side, making this Split another variant of Press.

Now, this is where Split gets even more interesting. In the above discussion, Split is considered as a way to move the energy in opposite directions and out opposing limbs, whether on different sides (both arms or a leg and the opposite-side arm) or on the same side (a leg and the same-side arm), or back together toward a center. But can this really be the core of Split? If the Cardinal Energies move the energy along specific planes, and the Ordinal Energies train coiling and twisting, then we can't think of Split as just moving the energy in two directions along a specific plane. We also must also find a coiling or twisting component at its core.

To find this necessary component, let's look back at the basic Split examples given at the beginning of this chapter: open Split, where the arms separate, and its

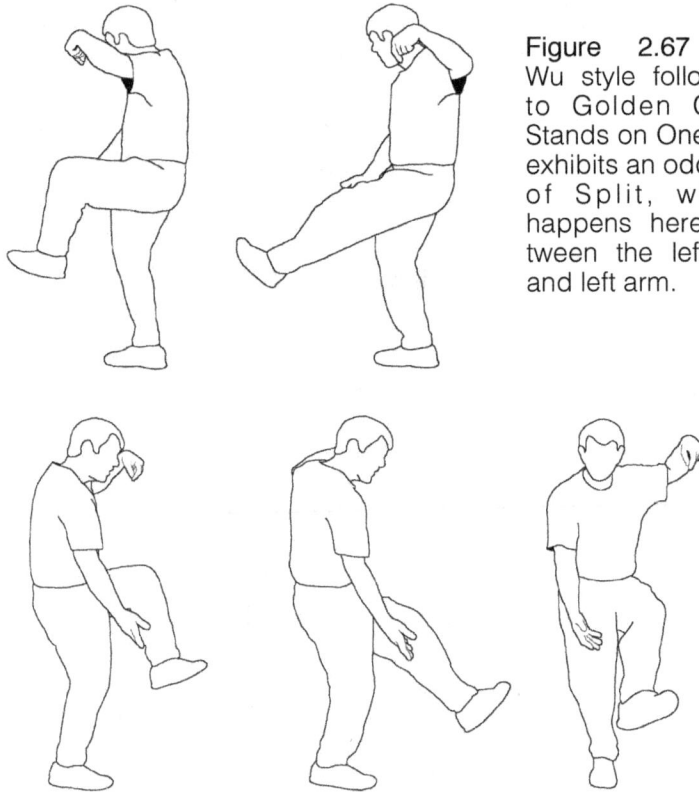

Figure 2.67 This Wu style follow-up to Golden Cock Stands on One Leg exhibits an odd use of Split, which happens here between the left leg and left arm.

yin equivalent, closed Split, where the arms come together. (Figure 2.68) Repeatedly going back and forth from open Split to closed Split twists the torso around Central Equilibrium, shaking the arms open and closed. But to avoid double-weighting, you can't just open and close both arms simultaneously and with equal force because, if you do, then you're trying to push off of both legs at once. This isn't really possible without resulting in torso and arm movements that are divorced from the hips and waist and are not only devoid of torque, but also use muscular upper-body strength rather than dynamic power. This is another perfect example of double-weighting and how this fault robs a movement of its power.

So, in order to open and close effectively and with power, one must first push the energy from one leg into the opposite leg, then rapidly push the energy from that leg back into the first leg, and so on, back and forth This causes the waist to do a slow-

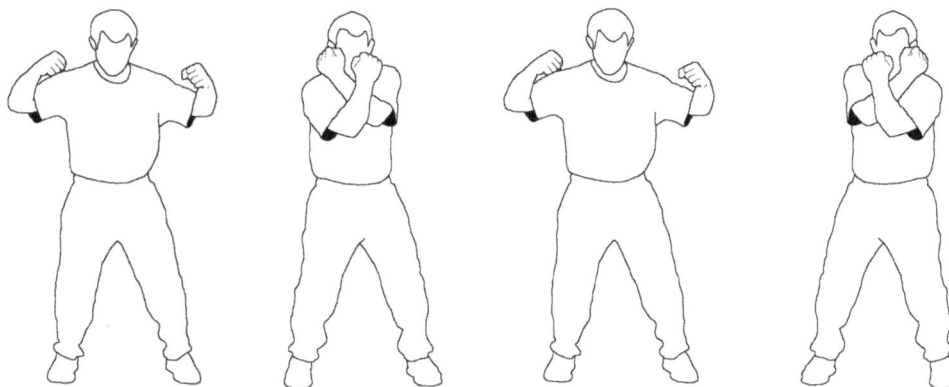

Figure 2.68 Repeatedly going back and forth from open Split to closed Split uses alternate pumping of the legs to twist the torso around Central Equilibrium, shaking the arms closed and open.

motion version of the rapid twisting movement a dog uses to shake water out of its fur: a rapid, back-and-forth Roll Back movement of the waist and hips that coils, uncoils, and re-coils the torso. This allows the legs to properly power the movement and twist the waist to effectively transmit the power through the torso and into the arms in a rapid, alternating sequence. This twisting and untwisting lends torque to the diagonal plane of Ward Off or to the straight forward/backward plane of Press, adding a secondary whipping power to those energies. In the case of Push, of course, the rotational whipping cannot apply, but there are Push movements, such as Golden Cock, that do utilize Split by tapping into the sinking and rising of the body weight to compensate for the lack of Roll Back's transverse torque.

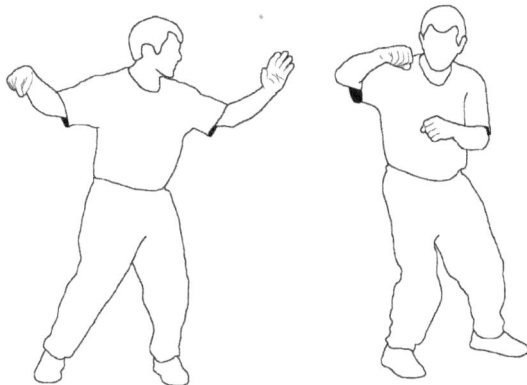

Figure 2.69 Single Whip's Split energy opens along the front of the body, while Beating Tiger's Split energy opens along the back of the body.

One can further differentiate the open Split as a pulling apart, as exemplified by Single Whip, or as a pushing apart, as sometimes exemplified by Beating Tiger. (Figure 2.69) Opening in these two ways feels different through the shoulders and back and directs the energy differently. The former uses the insides of the shoulders to send the energy through the insides of the arms and toward and into the hands, while the latter uses the outsides of the shoulders to accumulate energy in the outsides of the forearms, where it can be used, say, as an Elbow Strike with the forearm. This relates to the similar differentiation made in the previous section, where Pluck is energized from the same part of the shoulder as Single Whip, and Pull is energized from the same part of the shoulder as Beating Tiger.

Split works best with Ward Off and Press and less often with Push.

> If we desire to know the method of the circle, we must first find the correct point to issue from and the correct target, and then we will accomplish our task.
>
> —Wu Meng-hsia[13]

# Conclusion

**A couple of** examples of relatively simple relationships between the Cardinal and Ordinal Energies are Elbow Strike and Pull/Pluck, which similarly cause Press to ride the turn of Roll Back and could sometimes be considered the yang and yin aspect of the same movement. (Figure 2.70) Other combinations can be more complex. Single Whip, for example, can be thought of as a combination of Roll Back and Ward Off, using both Split and Pull/Pluck. (Figure 2.71)

So far, we've established the basic parameters of the pure forms of the Cardinal Energies and their functional blending to create the Ordinal Energies. We also looked at how and why the Ordinal Energies train the body to turn, twist, and coil. Now, let's look at the dynamics—first physical, then energetic—that alter the pure circles of the Cardinal Energies into martially effective movements.

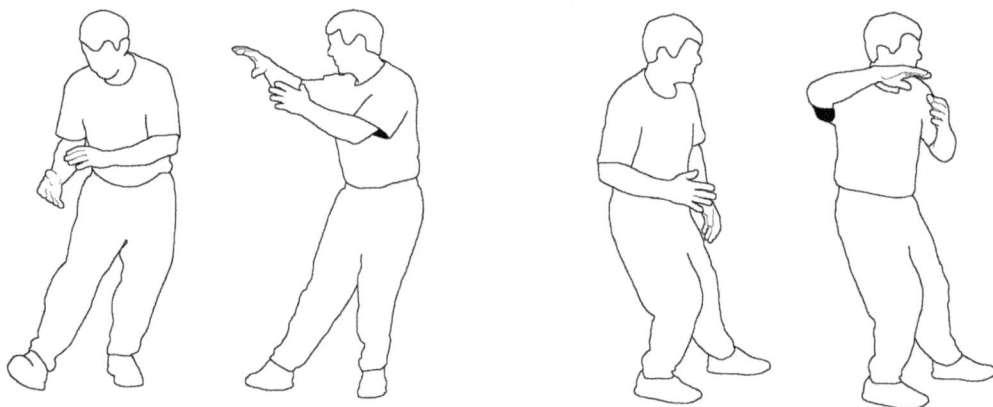

Figure 2.70 Pull/Pluck (left two) can sometimes function as a yin version of Elbow Strike (right two).

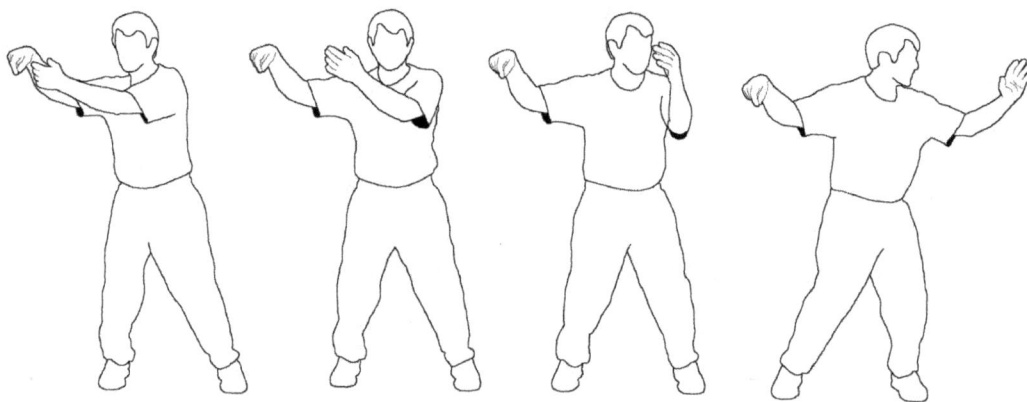

Figure 2.71 Single Whip combines the Cardinal Energies of Roll Back and Ward Off with the Ordinal Energies of Split and Pull/Pluck.

# ③ Symbol and Movement

Seek the curved in the straight, the straight in the curved; store first and then issue.

—Yang Lu-chan[14]

**Tai Chi is** renowned as a superlative martial art. Its foundation is the dynamics of the Thirteen Postures, though a number of factors enter into the mix that aren't directly related to the Thirteen Postures. I'll discuss some of those later, but to begin with, I want to continue the examination of the four Cardinal Energies and how the pure circles of each are transformed into martial force. In general, the pure circles of each Cardinal Energy can't be used martially. An exception might be to use the large Press circle by rotating the arm backward around the shoulder, motivated by a circling of the same-side hip, to redirect an incoming punch. In most cases, however, the pure circles have to be altered.

Let's not forget during this discussion that all arm movements are motivated by the feet and legs, directed by the waist, and transmitted through the torso, and only then are manifested in the arms. In a sense, Tai Chi movements are like a those old Saturn rockets used to propel the Gemini and Apollo capsules into space: The legs are the main booster, the waist is the guidance system, the torso is the secondary booster, the arms are the third-stage booster, and the hands are the capsule, or payload. The payload can't get into space without being lifted there through a sequential firing of each booster in turn, and being pointed in the correct direction by the guidance system.

Tai Chi's movements also can be looked at as containing a principle of folding and unfolding—a process of folding each joint in succession to absorb and redirect energy or, conversely, of unfolding each joint in succession to deliver energy. This makes of the body a sort of spring or shock absorber that compresses to receive incoming force then decompresses to expel the force outward. The way the Tai Chi Classics put it is that "one must learn to thread the energy, unbroken, through a pearl with nine bends or passageways"—the "Nine-Channel Pearl." In other words, we must direct both physical force and chi power sequentially through the nine joints from ankle through the last joint in the fingers: ankle, knee, hip, shoulder, elbow, wrist, first knuckle, second knuckle, and third knuckle.

I'll look at this again in later sections. For now, though, it is too unwieldy to explicate every facet of every movement in the descriptions that follow, so I'll generally forgo descriptions of the sinking or settling of the weight then the subsequent thrusting of the legs to power the waist, etc., through the sequence of joints and their associated muscle and tendon groups, taking them for granted until we discuss them later in more depth.

> The Tai-Chi is not only a circular plane figure in a still condition, but also a moving object like a rotating globe.... One may observe that the Tai-Chi diagram accurately represents the circular motion of various objects, from whirlpools to spiral nebulae.
>
> —Jou Tsung Hwa[15]

# Circles to Ovals

**The first step** in creating martial force out of the pure circles of the Cardinal Energies is that the circles have to be flattened into ovals. (Figure 3.1) Tai chi exponents are familiar with what are sometimes called the "long force" and the "short force." Most Tai Chi movements offer applications that execute either the long or short force, depending on purpose, need, or circumstance. Both utilize whole-body power, but in somewhat different ways. The long force is a powerful surging that repels or bounces an opponent away, and the short force is a sharper jolt that penetrates

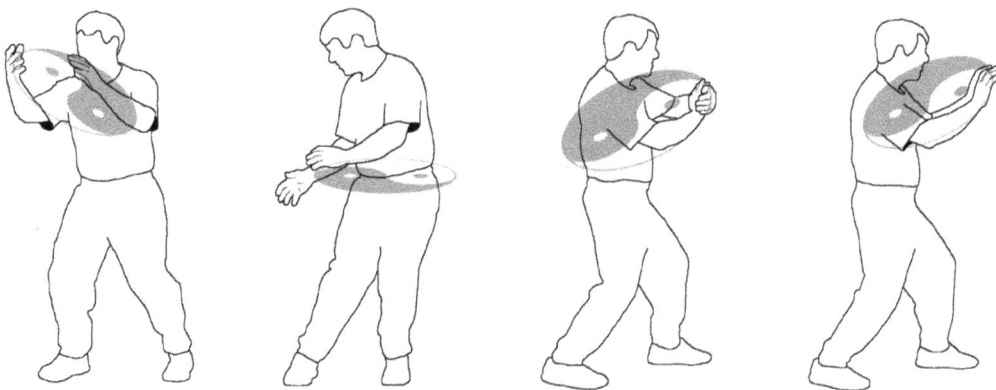

Figure 3.1 To make the circles of the four Cardinal Energies martially effective, they must be flattened into ovals. Left to right: Ward Off, Roll Back, Press, and Push.

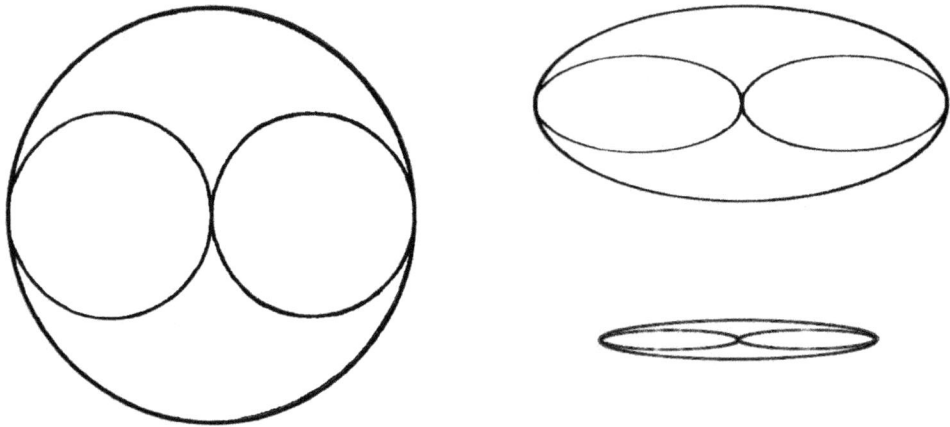

Figure 3.2 Flattening a Cardinal Energy circle produces greater force around the pointed ends. The flatter and shorter the circle, the shorter and more penetrating the force becomes.

the opponent or wrenches his limb. Both of these abilities are examples of fa jin, the ability to apply a wave of force to the opponent for the purpose of defense or offense, but they differ in the quality of the energy they deliver or receive.

Think of Push. You can use it to shove an opponent away, often lofting him to some distance, without doing him much direct harm, or you can use it to shock his internal structure, potentially damaging organs or breaking bones. The energy you use is the same in both instances, but the difference lies in how much you flatten the Push circle. In the case of the long force, you flatten the circle only slightly, and in the short force, you flatten it to a greater degree. (Figure 3.2) Using long and short force is possible even with Roll Back, which might seem to be lacking in issuing force. The flatter the Roll Back oval, the more suddenly and precipitously the opponent is led into emptiness. Also, any follow-up by the trailing hand, such as an elbow lock or break, is likewise sharper.

Flattening the pure circle into an oval alters not just the circle's shape, it also affects the duration of the movement. The duration of the long force is greater than that of the short force. Hence, the long force is long because it isn't just longer in a physical sense—stretched out—but because it occurs over a longer span of time than the short force. The oval of the short force is not just flatter and shorter in distance traveled, but it takes a shorter in time. The general principle here is that the flatter and smaller the

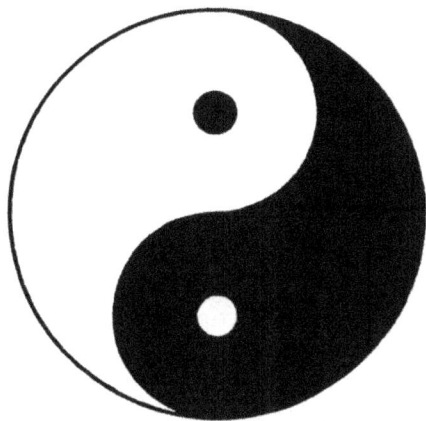

Figure 3.3 The tai chi symbol is one of the most recognized images in the world.

oval, the shorter, quicker, and more penetrating the force.

One of the elements of Tai Chi mastery is not only to be able to execute any given Cardinal Energy as a long force, but also as a short force. And the smaller the oval of a short force, the more invisible the technique is to onlookers—one reason for the seemingly miraculous abilities of great masters to defeat opponents without appearing to move much at all. Moreover, deep mastery is the ability to use the short force in a gentle manner as well as in a jolting one. I think here of the several videos of aged master Wu stylist Ma Yueh-liang bouncing around his much younger push hands opponents with barely a touch. Master Ma had developed his short force to such a refined state that the ovals of his movements were not only incredibly small and short but also incredibly focused and controlled in their delivery of energy.

But turning circles into ovals and shortening their length and duration aren't the only factors at play. To examine what might be the most important element, let's look at the tai chi symbol, which, if the story of Ong Tong He related in the "Introduction" is true, is the origin of the very appropriate name of the art. To remind you: Ong witnessed the great and undefeated Yang Lu-chan in action and wrote, "Hands holding Taiji shakes the whole world, a chest containing ultimate skill defeats a gathering of heroes."[16] What was it Ong saw in Yang's art that caused him to think of the tai chi symbol?

The tai chi symbol is well-known almost the world over as a representation of Taoism. It is, in fact, one of the most profound symbols to be found on the planet—a profoundness belied by its visual simplicity: a circle evenly divided by a symmetrical wavy line, one side colored white and the other black, each side decorated in mirror image with a spot of color opposite that of its own composition. (Figure 3.3)

The symbol implies the duality of all the universal conditions, forces, impulses, and states known in reality: forward/backward, male/female, up/down, hot/cold, on/off, good/evil, attack/retreat...the list is practically endless. The tai chi symbol also can symbolize the bifurcated mind—the left/right, rational/intuitive brain—with two eyes staring into the world—or into itself. It also is, as I discussed in *The Wellspring*, a very interesting visualization of the physiological aspect of the chi's circulation through the body. It is as well, as mentioned earlier, a representation in two dimensions of our four-dimensional reality: the circle implies a sphere, and the wavy line implies spin, or motion over time.

For Tai Chi enthusiasts, the tai chi symbol represents the basic martial aspect of Tai Chi in its alternation of yin and yang: the constant shifts of yielding and issuing power, both of which ideally occur in perfect and balanced conjunction. But the relationship of the two goes much deeper. For our purposes here in discussing Tai Chi as a martial art, the tai chi symbol opens the door to the way the pure circles, altered into flattened ovals, transform the four Cardinal Energies into martially useful power.

The way though this door lies in studying two opposing forces (surprise!) that we know from physics: the yang of centrifugal force, which is the force that tends to impel an object outward from the center of rotation, and the yin of centripetal force, which is the force that is necessary to keep an object moving in a circular path and that is directed inward toward the center of rotation. Let's forget for a moment that science considers centrifugal force to be a false, or virtual, force—really, it's just a lack of centripetal force. But virtual forces can exist within accelerating bodies, and in a rotating system the virtual centrifugal force is away from the center.

Centrifugal force, unchecked—or, conversely, under very controlled circumstances—will fling away an incoming force. Centripetal force, unchecked—or, again, under very controlled circumstances—will pull incoming force inward. (Figure 3.4) We are familiar with these forces as they affect planetary bodies. Planets orbiting the sun do not fall into the sun's gravitational well because centrifugal force —angular momentum—keeps them moving away from the sun. Likewise, they are not flung into deep space despite their momentum because centripetal force, or the force of gravity, keeps pulling them inward. A planet with a stable orbit exhibits perfect balance between these two forces.

Both centrifugal force and centripetal force are implied in the tai chi symbol, the former in the peripheral circle and the latter in the curved central line. But it is the recurved nature of that central line that is significant, along with the idea that yang is constantly changing to yin and yin to yang, for the line is what provides a path to smoothly transition from yang to yin and back again—smooth in the sense that the force does not have to stop to change direction but can transform into its opposite without pause or angular change.

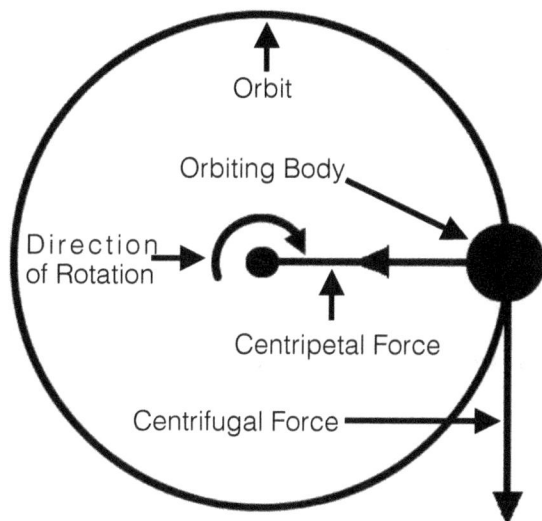

**Figure 3.4** Centripetal and centrifugal forces at work in a dynamic rotational system.

It is in the moment of change from yang to yin and yin to yang that Tai Chi's power manifests. As pure yang force swinging around the outside circle transforms into yin, it dips inward toward the inside of the circle until it reaches the center of the circle, or, the pure yin state. At this point, the pure yin force begins to arc along the recurve, back toward the circumference, becoming, in the process, yang force and also reversing the direction of the circle's spin. (Figure 3.5) It it somewhat like that old logic problem: How far can a bear run into the woods? The answer is not: All the way through. It is: Half way, because after that, the bear is running out of the woods.

The point to note about the way the yang and yin forces change as they move through this configuration is that the circular, expansive yang force tightens up and condenses as it curves inward, creating a considerable compression of energy. Think of an ice skater performing a spin. The skater skates along in a straight line then suddenly stops and perches on the toe end of one skate and begins spinning. As she spins, she draws in her arms, which compresses the angular momentum into a tighter and tighter spin that increases dramatically in speed. An elite skater can complete an astounding average of six rotations per second and about seventy rotations per spin.

Let's call this compression of energy an exponential increase in the force because the power increases exponentially rather than in a simple linear (arithmetic) progression—the closer the skater pulls in her arms, the progressively faster she spins. Another example of exponential force is a phenomenon familiar to anyone who drives a car. You're driving along, and then you apply the brakes. If you apply a light, steady pressure, the car will come to a gradual halt. You might be pressed into your

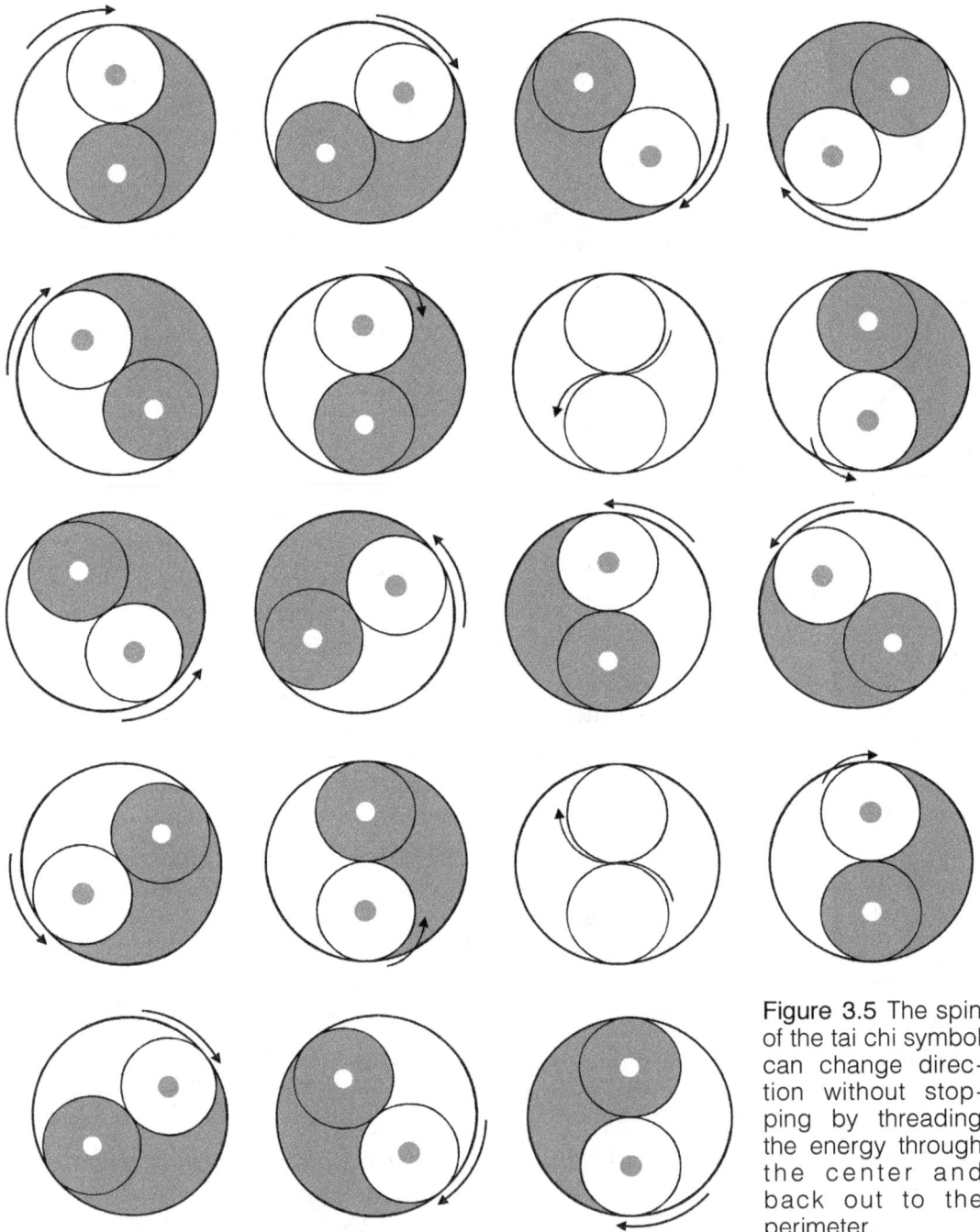

**Figure 3.5** The spin of the tai chi symbol can change direction without stopping by threading the energy through the center and back out to the perimeter.

shoulder harness, but the pressure will be light and steady. This is an example of linear deceleration. But if you put your foot on the brake pedal and apply intensifying pressure, the brake pads will grip with increasing strength, and the car will come to a sharply decelerating, screeching halt, throwing you into the shoulder harness with greater and greater force. This is an example of exponential deceleration.

Due to the rapidly increasing inward turn of the tai chi symbol's curve, the compression (located in the middle of the blank symbols in Figure 3.5) is not a simple linear deceleration but exhibits instead a progressively rapid deceleration and is thus exponential in nature. When the force reaches its ultimate compression at the center of the symbol, it, like the bear, can only begin to move outward. As the densely compressed yin force curves outward, it expands—again, because of the curve, which now opens outward—with exponentially increasing acceleration. Circling exponentially inward from the peripheral circle releases yang jin and produces yin jin, and circling exponentially outward releases yin jin and produces yang jin.

So, the recurved line that separates the two halves of the tai chi symbol points to a way to quickly and powerfully store and release energy. The Tai Chi exponent moves his energy (force and chi), backed by the momentum of the entire body, along an arc around the peripheral circle/oval of a Cardinal Energy, then suddenly changes the direction of the energy's trajectory by pulling it backward or pushing it forward (depending on whether the movement is yang or yin), around one or the other head of the recurved line. At the instant the energy begins to round the head of the recurve, it reaches its maximum possible acceleration/deceleration and power, and at this point, the exponent abruptly releases the energy of the movement, not by forcibly halting it, but by simply letting go of it. This causes the limb carrying the energy to recoil a short distance further around the recurve, but because a great deal of momentum has built up behind the movement, the energy of the movement continues in a straight line and is released into the opponent in the case of yang force, or away from the opponent in the case of yin force.

Figure 3.6 shows this in an aspect of Ward Off, but the principle holds true for any yang or yin movement around any of the Cardinal Energy ovals, and it is this rapid, exponential acceleration and deceleration around the heads of the recurves that gives Tai Chi movements their characteristic whipping/jerking motion.

The idea that the energy can leave the moving hand and continue on through space, at least for a short distance, might strike some as being rather esoteric. But is it? Tai Chi's whipping/jerking motions contain the same dynamics as the cracking of a whip, in which the whip-wielder sends a wave of energy down the flexible

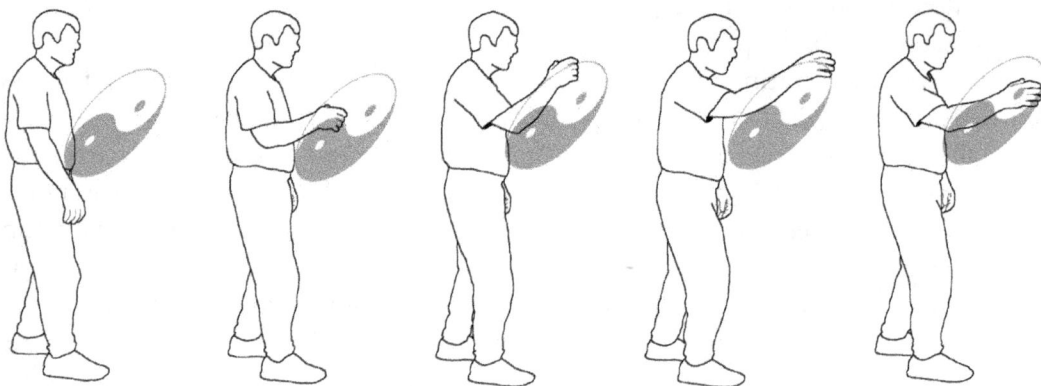

**Figure 3.6** The Ward Off arm sequence showing the energy moving forward around the head of the yang fish then recoiling inward: over the top of the oval (above) and under the bottom of the oval (below). The same motions occur when pulling the energy backward around the tai chi symbol.

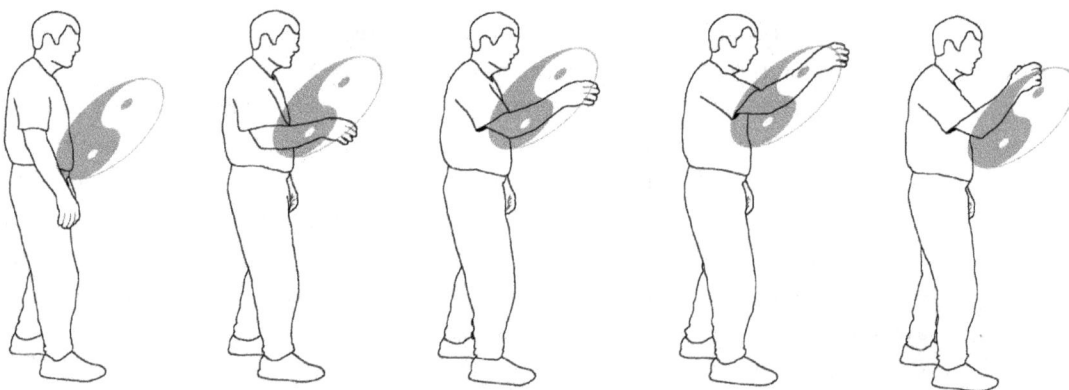

curve of the whip then suddenly pulls or jerks back on the handle and pauses. These combined actions cause the tip of the whip that is arcing around the head of the last curve—the head of the yang part of the tai chi symbol—to abruptly draw back then stop. The more abruptly the whipper jerks back and pauses, the sharper the resulting energy release when the tip rounds its final curve and snaps back. You can hear the energy of the whipping motion being released as an audible crack, and that same energy can do significant damage as it is snapped straight off the tip of the whip and into its target. (Figure 3.7) In Tai Chi, the whipping can be blunt or sharp —it all depends on how much you flatten and shorten the circles of the Cardinal Energies into ovals. An only slightly flattened oval will produce a blunter force, and a highly flattened oval will produce a sharper one—again, the long and short forces.

Let's look at an illustration from the physical world of how one can "ride" the yang energy, which has an interesting correlation to the fact that the two sides of the tai chi symbol resemble bent teardrops whose tails are curved. These bent teardrops are sometimes referred to as "fish" for their resemblance to that creature.

Fish inhabit water, and the power of Tai chi has often been equated with the force of water. The Tai Chi Classics state: "No force is softer or more penetrating than water, yet none is more powerful." For the latter aspect, don't think of a flood, which can be either a chaotic, rushing churn or a slowly rising inundation. Think instead of waves breaking on a beach, and put yourself inside the wave, as a surfer does when the wave breaks overhead and the surfer is then riding inside the "tube."

The tube, formed of a highly organized, uprising, and powerful wall of water, arcs overhead, then, as it completes its upward sweep and falls forward, the force becomes disorganized and dissipates—yang to yin. And the tube in which the surfer rides is not circular in shape but is shaped like a warped teardrop—like one of the tai chi symbol's fish. (Figure 3.8) Once the water of the wave arcs overhead, it is no longer backed by the energy that created its upwelling, and its yang state instantly evaporates into a passive yin state. The surfer merely rides the wave's upwelling yang energy for as long as the wave lasts.

However, this only relates to a surfer who wants a long ride as opposed to one who prefers to perform aerial acrobatics by jumping his board over the lips of breaking waves. Any breaking wave consists of the yang upsweep, though many waves, particularly early on in their breaking, don't actually form a tube. But this gives the surfer an opportunity that a tube doesn't offer because even without tub- ing, the lip of the wave is the moment where the force of the wave around the head of the yang fish suddenly dips inward into the recurve, changing to yin and gaining

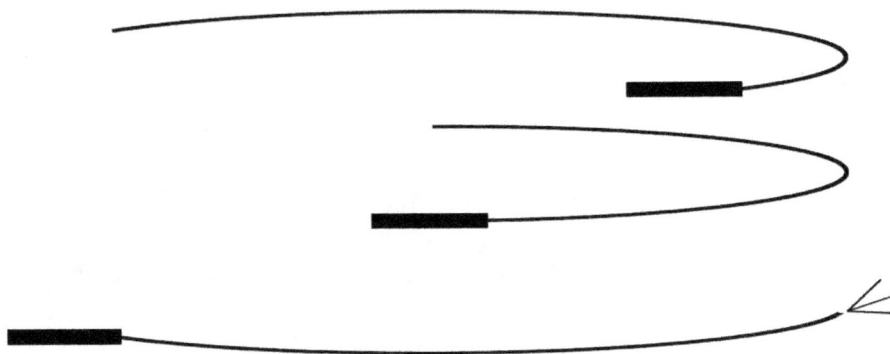

Figure 3.7 When a whip is pulled sharply around a curve then jerked back, it sends energy off its tip with an audible cracking sound.

a sudden final burst and release of energy. It just doesn't show a visible manifestation. This is the point at which acrobatic surfers can tap into the full strength of the yang uplift to propel themselves into the air to do spins and flips, leaving the propelling force of the water behind. They are taking advantage of the same energy that snaps off the tip of a whip, the same energy that the Tai Chi exponent uses when he whips his limb around the head of the yang fish then suddenly relaxes it, causing the energy of the movement to continue on in a straight line.

In fact, all natural actions involve resistance followed by a deeper swooping in as the inertia of stillness—a body at rest tends to remain at rest—is overcome by the inertia of movement—in the absence of friction, a body in motion tends to remain in motion. This probably happens at all levels, but at a basic physical level, it occurs as force overcomes friction: There is a momentary resistance, then a breaking free followed by increasing acceleration as long as the impelling force continues to accelerate. Once the impelling force ceases to accelerate, the energy dissipates—thanks to friction—and falls back into a steady state.

In physical confrontation, this friction is the momentary resistance that occurs when a person is pushed, which can be manipulated by Tai Chi movements—fa jin, for example, being a method to break the opponent's inertia of stillness (root) and follow that with a sudden swoop of energy that pushes, jolts, or otherwise manipulates the opponent. In fact, Tai Chi power is often likened to a wave of energy, force, or whole-body strength.

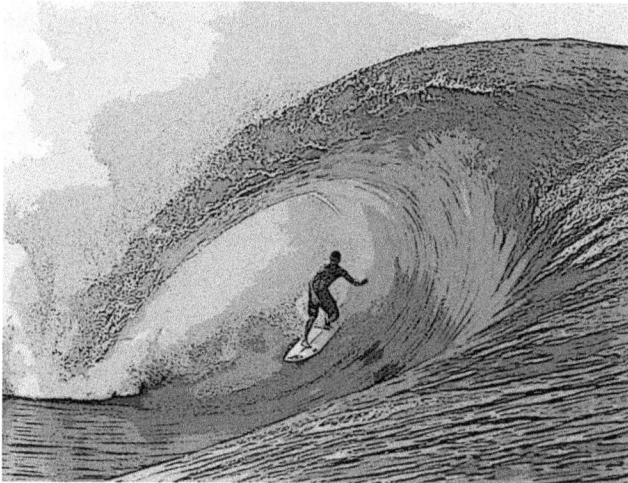

Figure 3.8 A breaking wave forms the bent teardrop shape of one of the fish of the tai chi symbol.

Theoretically, you could put emphasis on this energy just about anywhere you want to as it cycles around the circumferences of these circles, but due to the limits of human physiology, some arcs are more functional than others. It strikes me that perhaps the several main styles of Tai Chi differ primarily in the part of the tai chi energy loop they play. Yang stylists, for example, seem to predominantly use the swing downward then up, while Wu stylists and some others are more the up and over types. Chen seems to play the middle range, which makes sense as it is the first recorded style, so subsequent significant variations would have to concentrate in either going over the top or under the bottom.

I'm not familiar enough with the operations of Yang and Chen Styles, however, to verify or disprove this speculation at this time. But we can definitely relate the major styles to the size of the sphere/oval they play, which is directly reflected in what is often called a style's "frame size," or, the depth of the stance and breadth of movement used by those styles. Yang and Sun are large-frame styles that generally engage the opponent at a longer-ranges; Chen is a medium-frame style that engages the opponent in the middle range; while Wu and Hao are small-frame styles that engage the opponent at short-ranges.

When sparring with opponents, whether push-
hands or free-hand, no matter how we reckon it,
the principles are: the great circle, the small circle,
the half circle, the marvel of yin and yang, full and
empty in the feet, the T'ai-chi yin-yang fishes, and
maintaining vertical. Though we flow unceasingly
through myriad changes, the principles of T'ai-chi
remain the same.

—Wang Tsung-yueh[17]

# Chan-ssu Chin

**In Tai Chi,** the dynamic principles taught by the tai chi symbol are illustrated during the most basic form of Chan-ssu Chin, the Tai Chi "Reeling Silk Exercises." Originally, Chan-ssu Chin was an element of Chen style, but it can be applied to any style. It is called Reeling Silk Exercises because of its resemblance to the sensation of harvesting silk threads from the cocoon of the silk worm. One grasps the end of the thread and gently pulls the thread out farther and farther. The pulling must be steady, even, and constant: too light a pull, and the silk will not unreel from the cocoon, and a pull that is too strong or uneven will break the thread.

This description highlights what is one of Tai Chi's most important characteristics. Most people identify Tai Chi by its slow speed, but a more important attribute is its continuity of movement, which helps lead both force and chi smoothly throughout the body. Moving slowly has specific benefits, such as improving strength, balance, and timing and giving opportunity for observational awareness of the body and to make subtle corrections, among other things. But although Tai Chi is most commonly practiced at a fairly slow pace, it can be practiced at faster speeds, too, revealing information that is invisible at slower speeds. And Tai Chi's slowness of practice hasn't remained consistent over time. Observe, for example, old film footage of Tai Chi experts. Even the Yang stylists often move at a pretty good clip compared to their modern-day counterparts, but their movements are always smooth, flowing, and connected. And, of course, if you were to actually use Tai Chi for self-defense, you might move quite rapidly, but you would still need continuity of movement to execute the applications properly.

In Tai Chi, it is the continuity of the flow of the movements and chi that really counts. You should have a light but steady sensation of constantly pulling and pushing an internal force or energy through the various patterns of motion. In addition to training continuity, Chan-ssu Chin exercises create a greater awareness in one's body of the yin and yang forces and help teach one to apply

> Chan-Ssu Chin works like a screw, which transforms the motion from any force acting on its thread into a spiral pattern, because of the change in the radius of curvature at any place.
>
> —Jou Tsung Hwa[18]

them in directly practical ways. They also help teach whole-body power by causing one to use the entire body to move the hand and arm instead of moving the limbs independently of the body. There are many formalized styles and patterns of Chan-ssu Chin that utilize the various Cardinal and Ordinal Energies, and you also can do free-form Chan-ssu Chin based on Tai Chi movements or groups of movements. The purpose here is not to present an exhaustive catalog of Chan-ssu Chin forms but to illustrate the points made above through its most basic form.

In this most basic form, you stand with your feet about shoulder-width apart and use one hand or the other to trace the outlines of a large tai chi symbol in the air in front of your torso—or on a poster tacked to a wall. This tai chi symbol would have a diameter of the distance from your tantien to your chin. Using a poster is helpful for beginners, but it quickly becomes quite easy to visualize a tai chi symbol of the appropriate size in front of you. One major limitation to following a tai chi symbol on a poster is that the tai chi symbol depicts rotation in only one direction, whereas Chan-ssu Chin constantly switches the direction of rotation. A more useful poster would be a doubled tai chi symbol. (Figure 3.9A) A more serious limitation is that following the poster emphasizes the arm movement rather than the waist movement, which as we will see below, is the more important of the two.

The basic pattern of movement can be seen in Figure 3.5 on page 102, and the pattern as traced by the hand is illustrated in Figure 3.9B. First you circle one or the other hand in front of you in one direction for the desired number of circles, then you tighten the circle to arc around the head of the yang fish shape and toward the center. From there, the reverse arc around the head of the opposite fish takes your hand back to the circumference, though now going in the opposite direction than

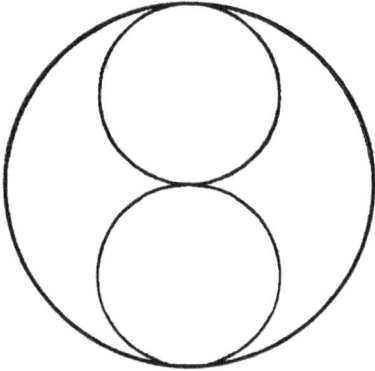

Figure 3.9A The doubled tai chi symbol is ideal to trace the basic pattern of Chan-ssu Chin.

before. After one or more revolutions around the periphery, the hand can follow another re-curve through the center, causing it to move in the original direction. Note that no matter which direction your hand is going around the circle, the circling inward along the recurved line always occurs around the head of the yang fish because that is where the energy is being released. The circling around the head of the yang fish can start at the top of the circle or at the bottom, depending on when you want to change direction, and both should be practiced with each arm.

The tai chi symbol traced by the hand is flat in front of you, but like a poster, it is really only on a secondary plane. Tai Chi is motivated by the legs and directed by the waist, so actually, the arm movement is merely a reflection of the rotation of a tai chi symbol on its primary plane, which is horizontal and bisects your torso at waist height, with the hips and waist using Roll Back alternating continuously from side to side to de-scribe the tai chi symbol around the central axis of the spine. We briefly talked about this sort of figure-eight waist movement in the discussion on Split. Note the waist-level tai chi symbol in Figure 3.9B. This is the symbol that you should actual-ly use to motivate the entire body movement, including the arm that traces the symbol in front of you. (Figure 3.10)

If you hold your arm loosely out in front of you and allow it to assume an elas-tic connection with your torso and then describe the figure-eight of the horizontal tai chi symbol with your hips and waist, motivated by alternate pumping of the legs, your arm will automatically follow the circling of the hip and waist movements but on the vertical plane. Simply rotating the hips in one direction or the other in a figure-eight pattern motivated by rhythmic pushes from one leg or the other will cause the hand on the opposite side from the pushing leg to describe the vertical tai chi symbol's outer perimeter, and the push from the predominant leg is what pro-pels the arm over the top of the vertical circle. The direction of the vertical symbol's rotation will be either clockwise or counterclockwise, depending on which leg is doing the pushing and which direction you are rotating your middle. If you are us-

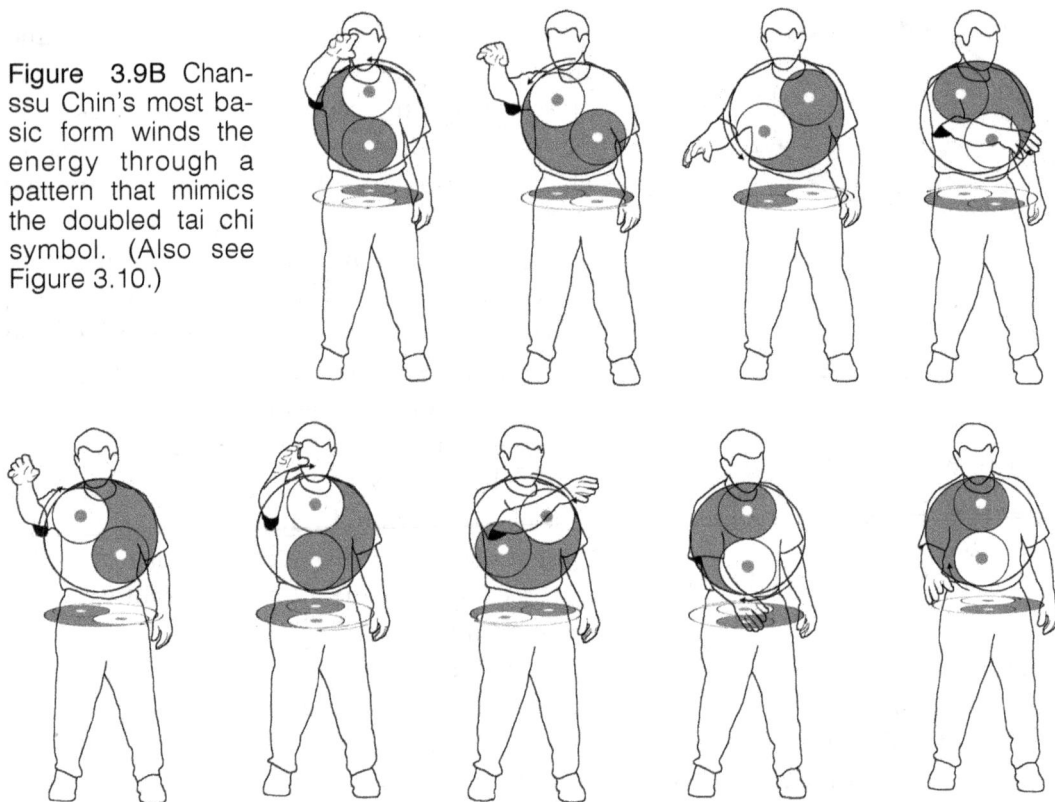

Figure 3.9B Chanssu Chin's most basic form winds the energy through a pattern that mimics the doubled tai chi symbol. (Also see Figure 3.10.)

ing your right arm, pushing predominantly with the left leg will rotate your arm clockwise, and pushing predominantly with the right leg will rotate it counterclockwise. The opposite is true for the left arm.

To change direction, you simply sink slightly onto the non-pushing leg when your weight goes onto it then begin pushing with it. This will propel the energy of the push in the opposite direction through the horizontal recurve and will cause the hips and waist to start circling in the opposite direction. It also will cause your extended, elastically connected arm and hand to automatically follow through the recurve in the vertical tai chi symbol you are creating in the air in front of you and return to the outer circle, also now going in the opposite direction. Swinging through the horizontal recurve again in the same fashion but in the opposite direction again reverses the direction of rotation of both horizontal and vertical symbols.

Note that the recurve of the tai chi symbol that is in front of you is oriented vertically at the moment of change, while the one that circles your hips is oriented side-to-

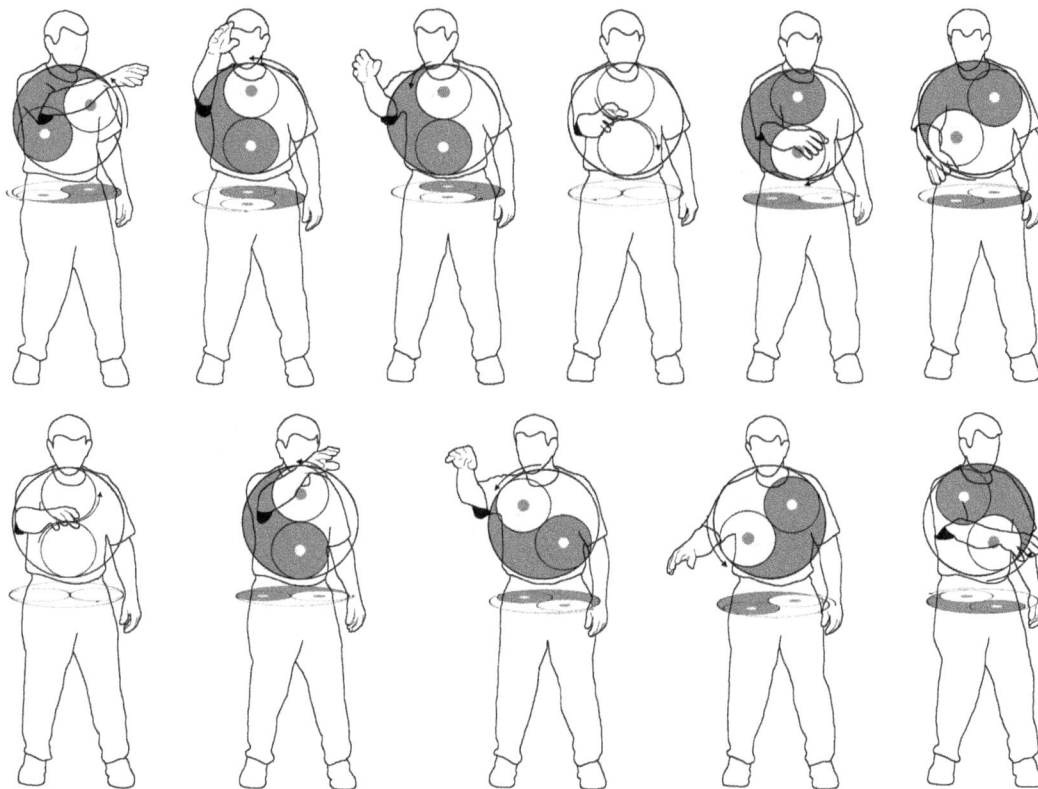

side. An interesting facet of the tai chi symbol formed by your hips and waist is that, if you take a bird's-eye view, whether you are circling or changing direction, the hip joints are where the eyes of the two fish are located. The smaller you can draw the symbol with your waist, the more refined and powerful your arm movements will be.

In many ways, this exercise does something similar to the one where you roll the Tai Chi sphere between your palms. (Figure 2.26, page 50) More important, you could say that this basic Chan-ssu Chin contains the distilled essence of Tai Chi, it just doesn't develop the permutations. Tai Chi's specialty is developing the permutations through training one to draw the physical force and energetic power through the Cardinal Energy spheres/ovals along various planes and with various twists and turns, using various stepping patterns, and in various combinations.

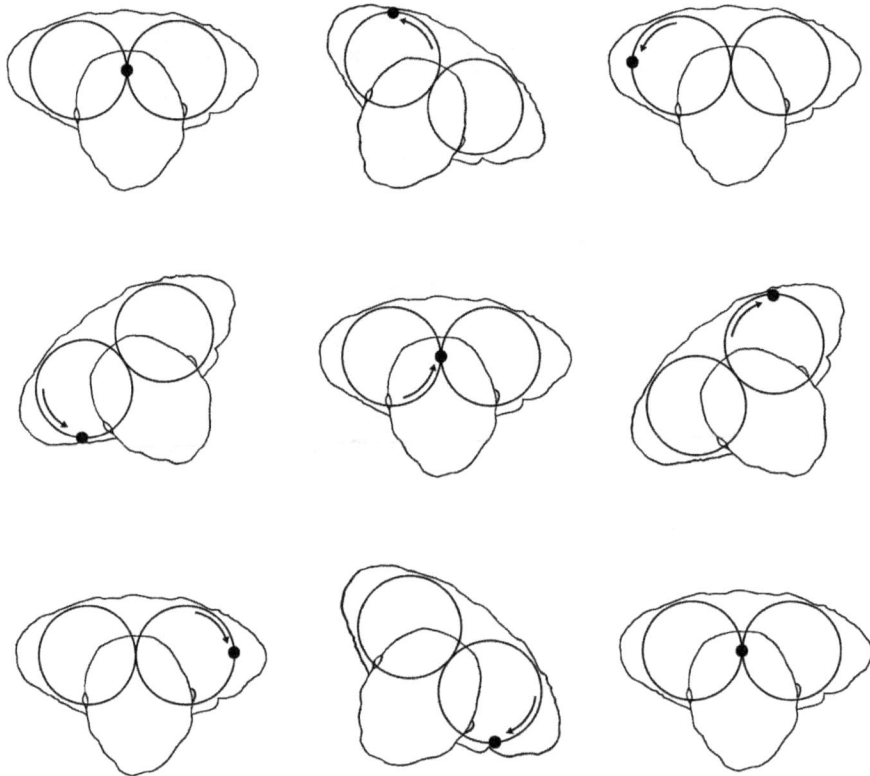

Figure 3.10 During Chan-ssu Chin, the primary plane of rotation is through the waist as you trace a figure-eight pattern, using your weight as a stylus. The arrow indicates the direction of movement, and the dot represents your sensation of weight.

# Power Emission

**Tai Chi's power** does not reside simply in the circles/ovals of the Cardinal Energies. The circles are the root elements, and flattening them into ovals increases their potential velocity and energy—the flatter the oval, the greater the uptick in both around the more sharply curved ends of the ovals. But it is in the curves and recurves depicted in the symbol that Tai Chi's real power lies. We looked at that in the previous section, but let's look closer still. Again, from the Tai Chi Classics: "Seek the straight in the curved and the curved in the straight." The "curved" is any curve embodied in the tai chi symbol, and the "straight" is any tangent that can issue from the spinning circle, either along its circumference or from any segment of its inner recurved line, as we saw previously. Let's start with the first half of this maxim—seeking the straight in the curved —in relation to the tai chi symbol and Tai Chi dynamics.

Yang force can be created in one of two ways. The first is to lead the force around the circumference of the symbol, toward the head of the yang fish, and then, at the apex of its reach, suddenly draw the issuing limb around the head of the fish, toward the center, and abruptly release it. The sudden dip inward, followed by release, exponentially increases the force's speed and power and transmits the force forward along a tangent outward from the the release point. (Figure 3.11) The second is to lead the movement, force, and energy through the second half of the recurved line, outward from the yin center toward the periphery, and suddenly release it, which also exponentially increases its speed and power and transmits the force backward along a tangent. In both cases, movement along a curved line abruptly alters to issue along a tangent— the straight in the curved.

Altering the curvilinear force that has been arcing around the perimeter into linear force is accomplished through use of a parabolic arc. A parabola is a two-dimensional, U-shaped mirror-symmetrical curve that can be in any orientation to its plane. (Figure 3.12) The arc of a parabola's arms, no matter how sharp or blunt its curve, does not circle back on itself. Instead, the arms open and extend infinitely.

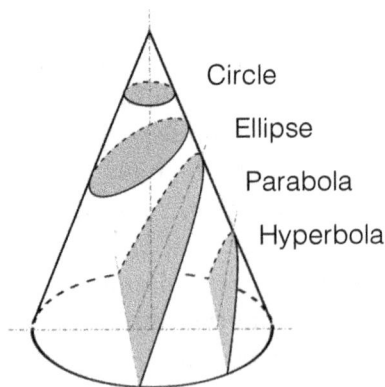

**Figure 3.11** Seeking the straight in the curved is the same as entering a tangent from a circular movement.

Strictly speaking, a parabola is a two-dimensional figure, but it often is utilized in three-dimensional forms, such as dish antennas, parabolic microphones, and light-gathering mirrors found in reflector telescopes. (Figure 3.13) In these instances, the three-dimensional object is called a paraboloid. The usual purpose of paraboloids is to gather weak incoming energy and focus it into a much more powerful and functional emanation: Think of an automobile headlight, which is a paraboloid that gathers the light from a relatively small bulb and focuses, and thus amplifies, the bulb's output into a cone-shaped beam of light that can effectively reach much more strongly in a given direction than light from the bulb alone.

The use of a sling shot is another real-world example of a parabola, and one that is martially oriented. I'm not talking about a forked stick with an elastic band, but the type use by David to kill Goliath, which consists of a leather pouch with a thong tied to each side.

The user places a stone in the pouch then grasps the ends of both thongs and whirls the stone in a circular motion above his head. At the appropriate moment, he suddenly releases one end of the thong, and the circularly whirling stone then goes flying

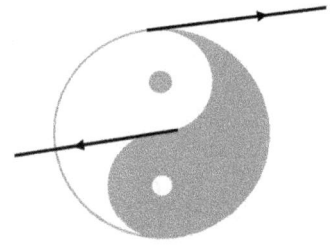

Circle
Ellipse
Parabola
Hyperbola

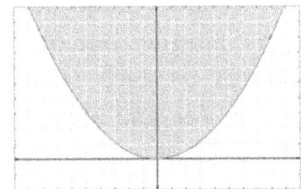

**Figure 3.12** A parabola is one of four conic sections. Its arms open up infinitely.

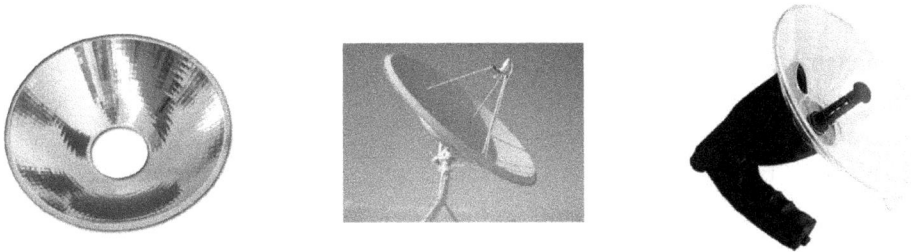

Figure 3.13 Paraboloids are used to focus relatively weak energy into a more powerful emanation. Left to right: light reflector, dish antenna, directional microphone.

in a straight line along a parabolic tangent. Yet another example is a jai alai ball being slung out of its basket. The ball goes from zero to about 120 miles per hour in less than a second because it is slung from its parabolic-shaped basket into a straight-line trajectory.

A similar method, called "gravity assist," is employed by NASA when its technicians use the gravity wells of planetary bodies to accelerate the velocities of exploratory space-craft, like the *Voyagers*, and fling them into deep space or to decelerate spacecraft returning to Earth. (Figure 3.14)

In many of its applications, Tai Chi takes advantage of something very much like a gravity assist, which is directly related to Tai Chi's torquing and which can dramatically increase Tai Chi's power. (Figure 3.15) In some cases, the issuing, or sometimes expulsive, force is created by drawing the energy

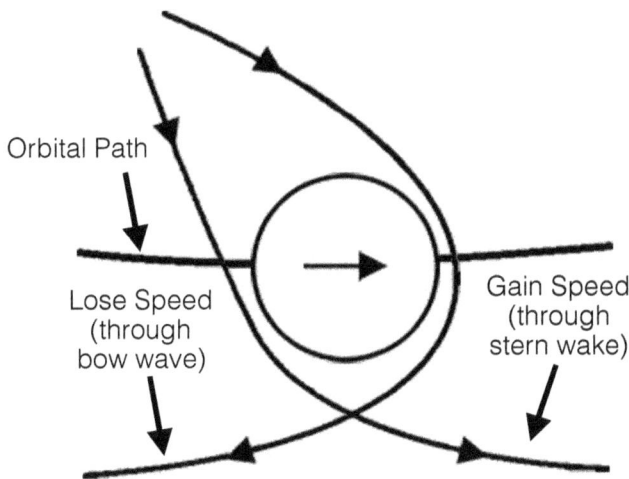

Orbital Path

Lose Speed
(through
bow wave)

Gain Speed
(through
stern wake)

Figure 3.14 NASA employs what is called a gravity assist, which uses planetary gravity to control orbital velocity to either speed up or slow down spacecraft.

through the parabolic arc, condensing it at the exact point of the arc, then issuing or expelling it. This is the "bumped away" trajectory in Figure 3.16 and is an example of Tai Chi's repelling power. The blunter the point of the parabola, the longer and more surging are the results; the sharper the point, the shorter and more jolting and penetrating they are. Both bluntness and sharpness refer to how much one flattens the Cardinal Energy circles into ovals.

There also is a somewhat more complex instance of finding the straight in the curved in Tai Chi. In this case, as the limb that carries the energy is rounding the apogee point of the yang fish head, it is pulled back abruptly around the inner curve of the yang fish head into a trajectory

Figure 3.15 Circling combined with rotation can allow Tai Chi movements to act like a gravity assist to speed up incoming energy.

that would intercept its original track if it kept going. However, as noted before, the moving limb stops before the energy actually crosses its original track. At the same time, at the exact point at which the hand starts to recoil into the recurve, the limb, formerly full of movement and energy, suddenly relaxes. This is the "flung away" path in Figure 3.16 and is one aspect of Tai Chi's whipping power.

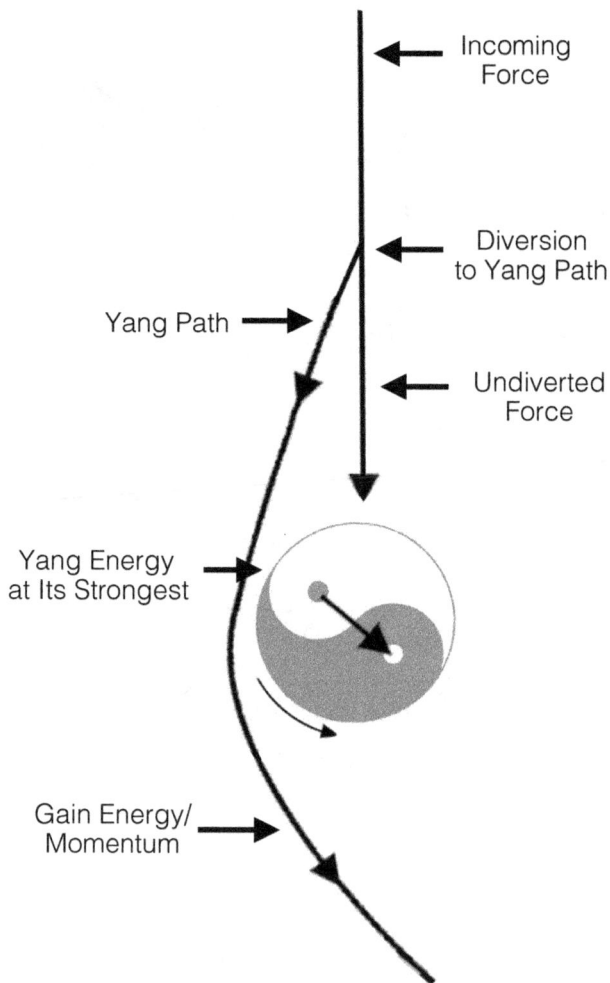

Incoming
Force

Diversion
to Yang Path

Yang Path

Undiverted
Force

Diverted Force
(Bumped Away)

Diverted Force
(Flung Away)

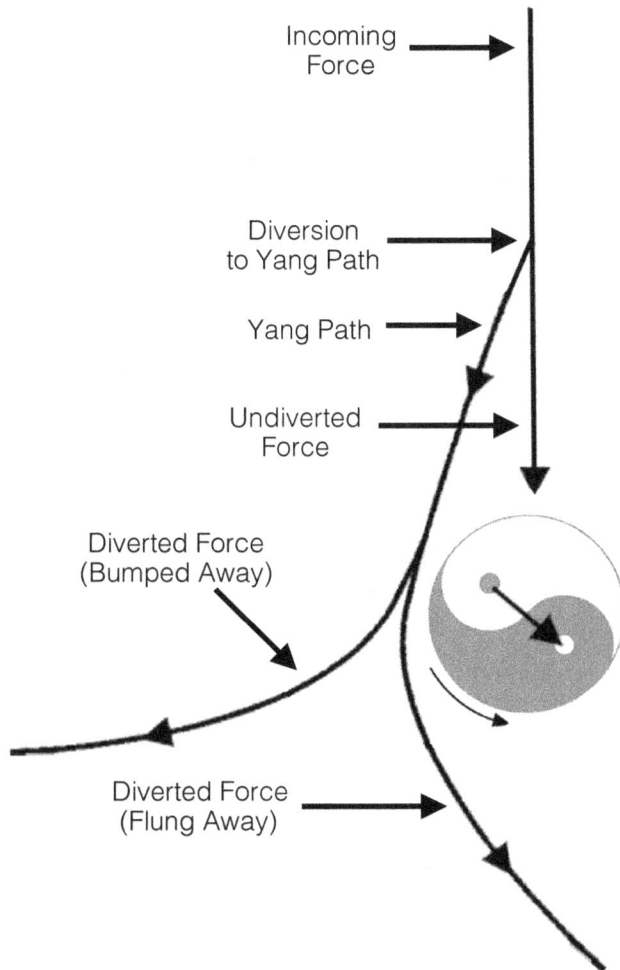

Figure 3.16 Along the yang path, incoming energy
can be diverted then either bumped or flung away.

In both cases, the moving hand describes the curve around the fish shape, but as soon as it passes around the yang fish's head and then relaxes and recoils from the yang apogee point, the energy it has been carrying can flow or surge past the apogee point and can be directed with considerable aim and force, either as a shove or strike or as a flinging movement. This is the same energy used to crack a whip or loft a surfer above the lip of a wave. And also in both cases, the infinite nature of the emanation—remember that parabolic arms extend infinitely without ever meeting—equates with the maxim from the Tai Chi Classics: "When I advance, my opponent feels as if there is no retreat."

Now let's look at the yin aspect of this: "seeking the curved in the straight." We can see that an incoming force, which usually has a straight line trajectory, can be diverted from its course by a relatively gentle sideways force. (Figure 3.17) This is because of the laws of inertia. The force (inertia of movement) of an energy moving in a straight line is highly directional, but from the side, there is no force at all. In fact, according to physics, the faster an

object moves, the lighter it becomes in all directions other than
the direction of its movement. In
Tai Chi terms, a fast-moving limb
is "floating" from any angle other
than the line of its trajectory. This
makes it easy to divert an incoming force with a relatively gentle
shove from the side. Two maxims
from the Tai Chi Classics address
this: "Four ounces defeats a thousand pounds," and "A simple error
in the beginning will result in a
deviation of a thousand miles."
The thousand pounds is the force
along the line of its trajectory, and
the four ounces is the light nudge
from the side that diverts the force

Figure 3.17 An object with directional force has no force in any other direction, so a relatively light pressure from any side can alter its trajectory.

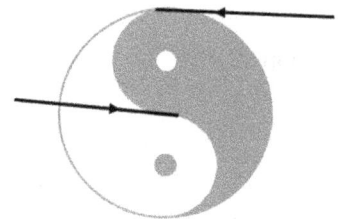

from its course. Once diverted, the force will miss its target because the angle of its trajectory has been altered, and the closer to its source that the force is diverted, the farther it will deviate from its original angle—the "thousand miles." In more familiar terms: A miss is as good as a mile.

Tai Chi's circular blocks tend to pull inwardly as well as nudge to the side, alter-ing the path of the incoming energy from a straight line into a parabolic track—

seeking the curved in the straight. This functions to
either send the force away along an ever-widening
angle of dissipating energy or to pull the incoming
force inward in a sharper and sharper arc, depending on the particular direction of the diversion. As
you can see in Figure 3.14, a gravity assist can be
used to slow down spacecraft as well as speed them
up. When the incoming energy reaches the center
point of the tai chi symbol's recurved line, the direction of the energy has been turned completely in
upon itself, rendering it not only useless, but giving
it the automatic potential either to be flung back-

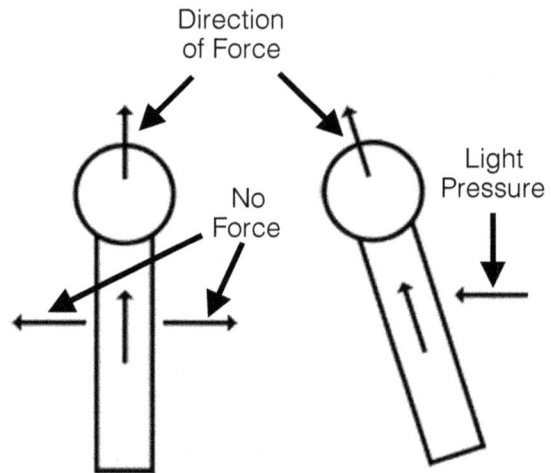

Figure 3.18 Seeking the curved in the straight is the same as entering a curve from a tangent.

Incoming Force

Diversion to Yin Path

Undiverted Force

Yin Path

Yin Energy at Its Strongest

Lose Energy/ Momentum

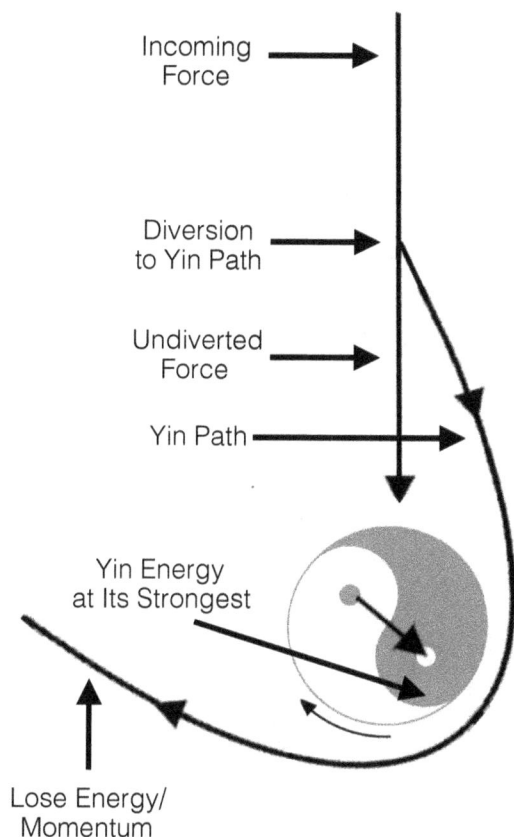

**Figure 3.19** Circling combined with rotation can allow Tai Chi movements to act like a gravity assist to slow down incoming energy.

ward or to be rebounded upon itself. Either can happen because not only does the energy of a gravity assist get manipulated around the symbol's periphery, it also occurs within each half of the recurved line, which form parabolic arcs of their own. (Figure 3.18)

But the incoming energy that is gathered by the parabola does not have to be just turned in on itself and slowed down. (Figure 3.19) A gravity assist also can put a spacecraft into a descending spiral. If one adds just a touch more inward energy to the side of an inward-curving parabolic arm, the touch of energy changes the path of the arm from a parabolic shape into a vortex, which sucks the energy inward into emptiness. (Figure 3.20) This would be the pure yin aspect reflected in the statement from the Tai Chi Classics: "If I retreat, my opponent is pulled deeper into emptiness."

Let's look at this another way. The straight-line aspect of incoming force also applies to straight-line retraction away from an incoming force. The difference is that while an attacking force relies on speed, strength, and power over a given distance, a direct retreat only requires speed over a given distance, although the speed must be slightly faster than the attacking speed, and the distance covered needs to be slightly greater in order to avoid the force.

But there is a way to increase both the speed and distance of a retreat by adding two additional dimensions to its retraction: turning and sinking. I mentioned this

Incoming
Force

Diversion
to Yin Path

Undiverted
Force

Yin Path

Diverted Force
(Sucked Inward)

Diverted Force
(Pulled Outward)

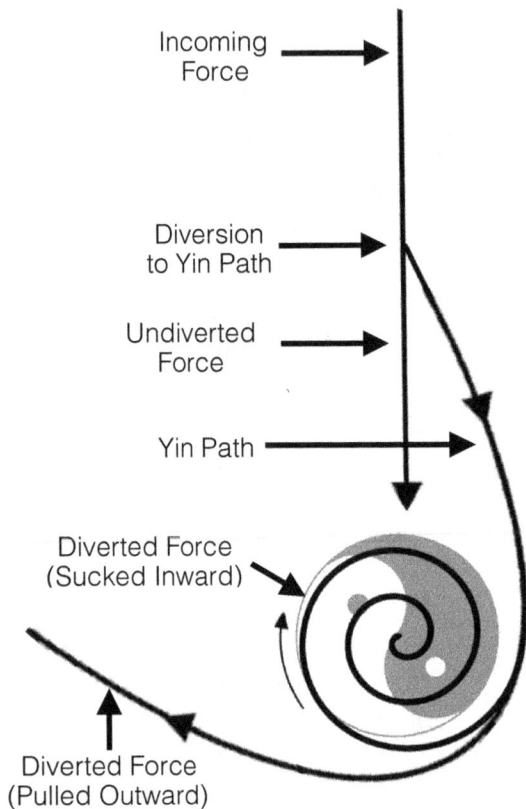

**Figure 3.20:** Along the yin path, incoming energy can be either diverted away outwardly or sucked inward.

same combination, although from a different angle, in the section on the Five Stances, referring to it there as a shift-twist-sink retreat. Turning and sinking while retreating instantly accomplishes several distinct but naturally interactive results. First, it immediately removes the defender from the direct line of the attack. Next, it changes the direction of the straight-line retreat without diminishing the retreat's speed. This abruptly lengthens the distance between the line of attack and its target—and in a shorter time—compared to the distance covered and time required by a straight-line retreat done alone. Third, it turns the defender's body to right angles (90°) to the attacker for optimal response against what is now his weak side. And finally, it automatically cocks the body for response, thus reducing reaction time. The net effect is to suck the incoming energy into a vortex that can be used to simply avoid the attacker's force, fling it away, or turn it back on him to cause him, say, to flip over or be slammed to the ground.

In fact, almost all Tai Chi movements that launch yang or yin energy directly use the parabolic arc and gravity assist. The arms can use a gravity assist upward, to the side, downward, or any angle in between. In general, the "gravity" in the arms is the physical attachment of the arms to the body. The waist can create a gravity assist horizontally by tapping into the rhythmic back-and-forth pumping of the legs. But the legs and torso tend to use a gravity assist by utilizing actual gravity, lowering the body weight in a downward arcing curve that then surges upward, propelled by the thrust-

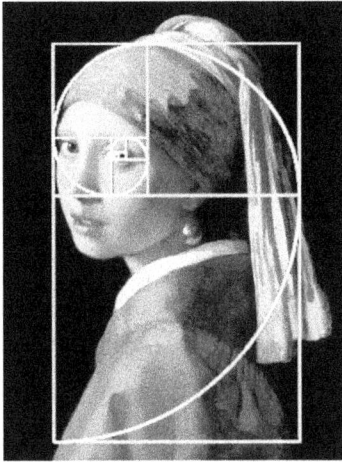

Figure 3.21 Johannes Vermeer's *Girl with a Pearl Earring.*

ing of the energetic leg. This also, as noted earlier, is how Push compensates for its lack of transverse torque. We'll look at that more later, but for now, it's important to note that the yang and yin aspects of the parabola and vortex are not generally separate but work together simultaneously.

Now, let's look at the tai chi symbol and the idea of spiraling inward and outward in a way that illustrates not only the functionality of Tai Chi but also its universal beauty. This has to do with a mathematical concept called the "golden ratio."

Mathematically, the golden ratio occurs when the ratio of two quantities is the same as the ratio of their sum to the larger of the two quantities. In other words, where $a$ is the larger quantity, there is a golden ratio if $a+b$ is to $a$ as $a$ is to $b$.[19] Mathematicians since Euclid have studied the properties of the golden ratio, and in 1202, the Italian mathematician Fibonacci (Leonardo Pisano Bigollo) published a sequence of numbers—called the Fibonacci Sequence—that approximate the golden ratio. This sequence has since found application in computer algorithms, graphs, and other scientific and mathematical techniques.

Indeed, the golden ratio also is called the "divine proportion" because it is exhibited in natural physical structures, such as the branching of trees, the arrangement of leaves on a stem, the fruit sprouts of a pineapple, the flowering of an artichoke, the uncurling of a fern, the arrangement of a pine cone, the veins of leaves, the spiral form of some mollusk shells, and many other instances. Adolf Zeising, whose main interests were mathematics and philosophy, found the golden ratio expressed in the skeletons of animals and the branching of their veins and nerves, the proportions of chemical compounds, and the geometry of crystals. The golden ratio's ubiquitous presence throughout nature prompted him to see it as a universal law of natural structure. In 1854, Zeising wrote that this universal law "contained the ground-principle of all formative striving for beauty and completeness in the realms of both nature and art, and which permeates, as a paramount spiritual ideal, all structures, forms and proportions, whether cosmic or individual, organic or inorganic, acoustic or optical; which finds its fullest realization, however, in the human form."[20]

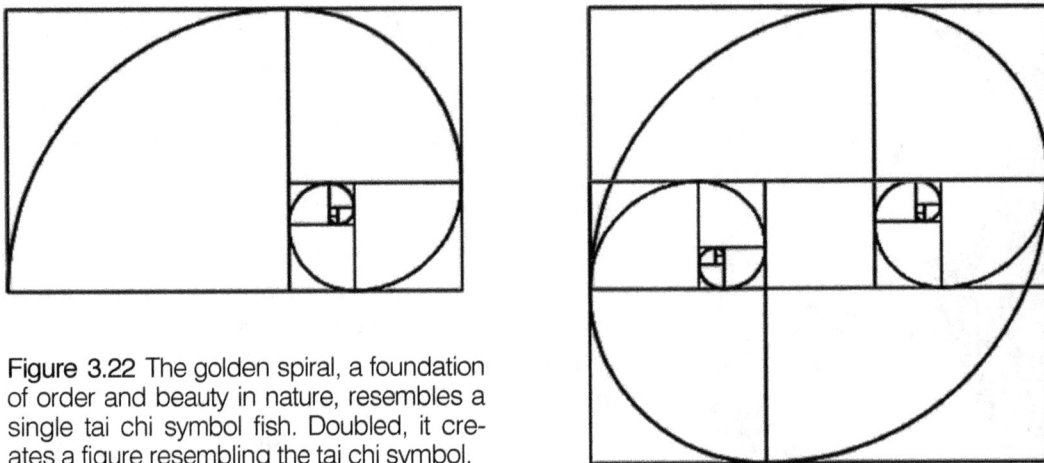

Figure 3.22 The golden spiral, a foundation of order and beauty in nature, resembles a single tai chi symbol fish. Doubled, it creates a figure resembling the tai chi symbol.

Naturally, artists as well as scientists and mathematicians have been fascinated with the golden ratio. An excellent example is *Girl with a Pearl Earring* by Johannes Vermeer (Figure 3.21), and it has been used more recently by Salvador Dali, Piet Mondrian, and others. The Argentinean sculptor, Pablo Tosto, has listed more than 350 works by well-known artists whose canvasses feature the golden ratio or a close approximation. It is found in the architecture of the Great Mosque of Kairouan, and the famous Swiss architect Le Corbusier extensively used the golden ratio in his designs. It also is present in the proportions of Medieval manuscripts, and even in music. Musicologist Roy Howat has observed that the formal boundaries of Claude Debussy's *La Mer* correspond exactly to the golden ratio, although it is disputed whether this was deliberate or not.

For Tai Chi enthusiasts, the golden ratio should have its own special meaning, particularly when it is converted, using the Fibonacci Sequence or other techniques, into a visual representation called the "golden spiral." The golden spiral is a logarithmic spiral that gets wider by a factor of the golden ratio for every quarter turn it makes. One look at this spiral (Figure 3.22), and you will instantly see what I mean. A single spiral is similar to one tai chi symbol fish, and when the spiral is doubled, it forms an approximation of the entire tai chi symbol—or, rather, the tai chi symbol approximates a doubled golden spiral.

The tai chi symbol, in its modern form, was developed in China, interestingly enough, at about the same time that Fibonacci was defining his mathematical sequence, but it has a history that goes back much farther. It also can be found in

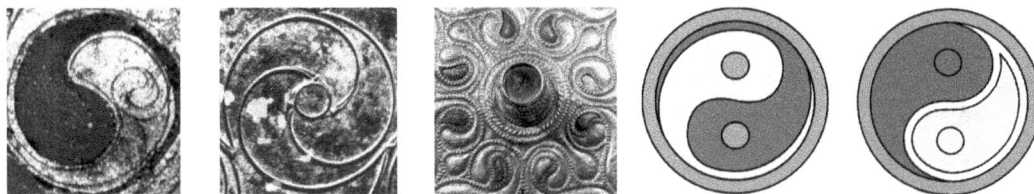

**Figure 3.23** Designs similar to the tai chi symbol have been used by different cultures through the ages. Left to right: three Celtic symbols (an ornamental bronze plaque from horse gear, a bronze disc, and a gold-plated disc) and two shield designs used by the Roman army.[21]

motifs of several Western cultures over the centuries, although there seems to be no direct influence by or upon the Chinese scholars who developed the Taoist version. (Figure 3.23) The tai chi symbol, it would seem, does carry profound and manifold universal meaning, which is no great surprise considering its resemblance to the golden spiral, and the basis of both in the golden ratio.

Figure 3.24 depicts how the tai chi symbol and the golden spiral can work together to illustrate Tai Chi's ability to draw incoming energy into a vortex and then expel it through an unwinding of the vortex. It also demonstrates the fact that Tai Chi, like the tai chi symbol, the golden spiral, and the golden ratio, is fractal: No matter what its scale, it always takes the same form and operates on the same principles.

I also encourage the reader to look up the following entries in *Wikipedia* to see other examples from science and engineering regarding the operation of energy through the tai chi symbol: "Cassini Oval," "Poinsot Spirals," "Spiric Sections," "Trammel of Archimedes," "Watt's Curve," and "Watt's Linkage." I've written about these examples in *Elements of Power: Essays on the Art and Practice of Tai Chi Chuan.* You might understand the science as little as I did, but the images are effective in demonstrating the universality of the energy transfer implied by the tai chi symbol. The first three show still images, but the latter three have very interesting animations of how energy can be manipulated and magnified by sending it through the tai chi symbol's curves or around the ends of elongated ovals.

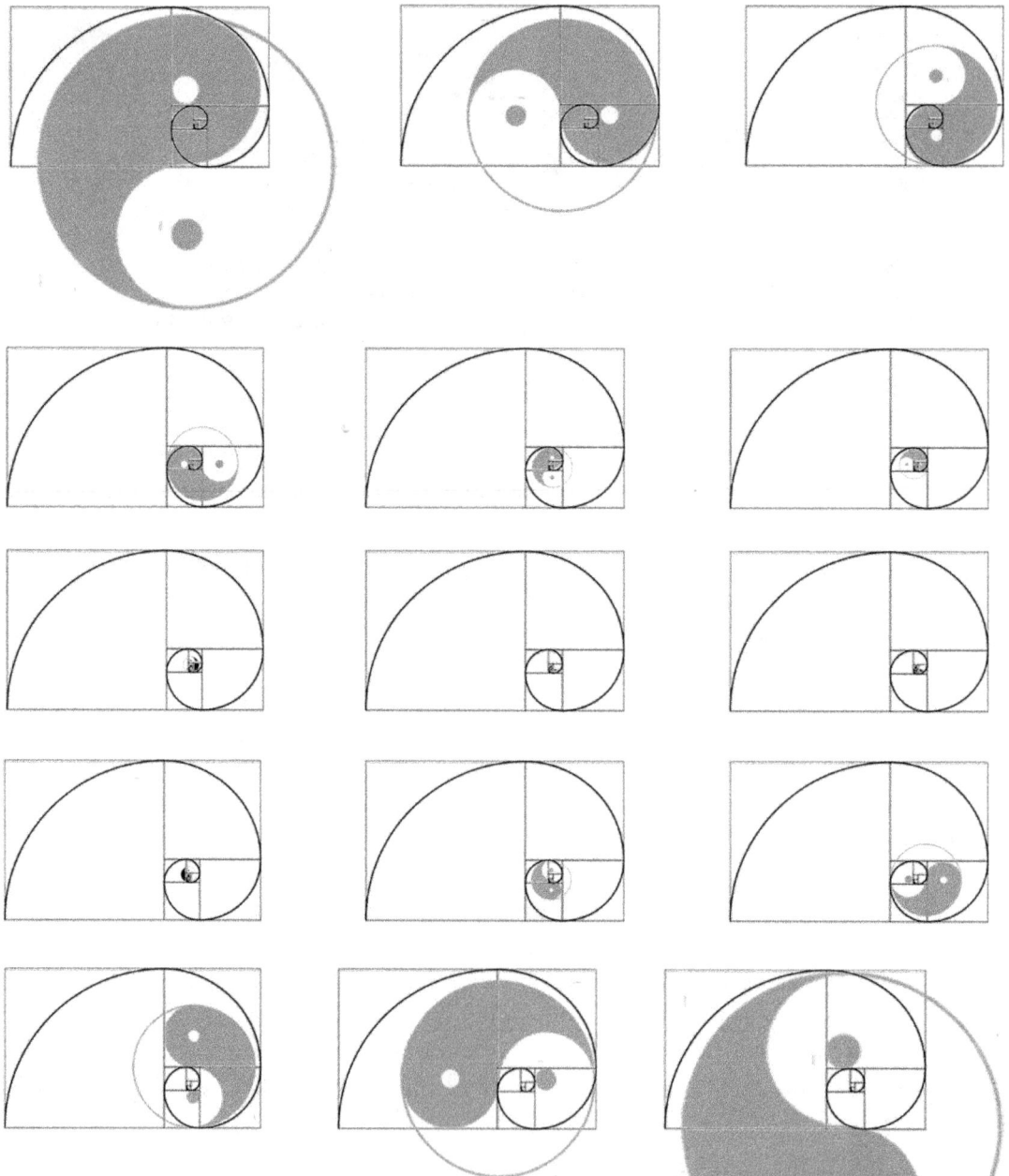

Figure 3.24 A combination of the tai chi symbol and the golden spiral demonstrates Tai Chi's ability to coil and then uncoil energy without halting its movement.

# ④ Breathing

**When I was** young—about five—I noticed that I was breathing differently than older people. My abdomen pooched out on my in-breath and went in on my out-breath, while older people's chests expanded and contracted instead of their abdomens. I must be doing it wrong, I thought, and I consciously changed my pattern—a mistake that took me several years to correct once I began to study Tai Chi. If only I could have known about the precept from the Tai Chi Classics, "Breathe like a baby," maybe I could have saved myself a lot of time and effort.

Correct breathing is absolutely essential for Tai Chi to work, either martially or for health purposes. In *The Wellspring*, I detailed the specific mechanisms of how correct breathing generates and strengthens chi and propels it through the body, so I won't go into that in depth here, though aspects of it will come up later. In addition, there are a number of specialized yogic breathing methods that I also won't cover—mostly because I do not know or practice them. Instead, I'll discuss three basic types of breathing, beginning with chest breathing. Then we'll look at the two main methods of abdominal breathing: natural abdominal breathing and reverse abdominal breathing.

Chest breathing is the kind of breathing I mistakenly imitated, as described in the opening paragraph above. It expands and contracts the lungs by action of the intercostal muscles of the chest, causing the chest to expand to pull fresh air into the lungs and to contract to expel stale air. Most people breathe from the chest, but the problems caused by this type of breathing are several. First, it causes a stagnation of air in the lower portions of the lungs because it does not fully expel the carbon dioxide produced by the body's metabolism. Second, it causes the chi to "float" in the chest rather than helping it sink into the tantien. This has the immediate effect of causing some level of perpetual agitation and nervous tension, and it also has deeper negative implications, not the least of which is that the lungs and the relatively thin chest muscles don't produce chi in the quantity that the tantien does, nor can chest breathing efficiently propel the chi

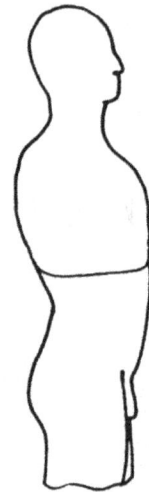

Figure 4.1 The diaphragm is a sheet of muscle between the lungs and viscera that controls breathing.

through the chi system. So chest breathing can't sufficiently generate or motivate chi, both of which are essential to good health as well as to Tai Chi's martial power.

Abdominal breathing works differently. Both types—natural and reverse—are motivated not by the chest muscles but instead by the diaphragm, which is a sheet of muscle that stretches through the abdomen below the lungs and above the viscera. (Figure 4.1) Most people, even if they breathe from the chest, are aware of the diaphragm when they get the hiccups, which are spasms of this muscle.

In natural abdominal breathing, all breathing—in and out—is done through the nose. The practice consists of breathing in by expanding the diaphragm evenly downward and breathing out by contracting it evenly upward, back into its relatively flattened shape. (Figure 4.2) Doing this on the in-breath sucks fresh air deeply into the lungs from the bottom rather than by pulling it in only at the top. On the out-breath, the diaphragm's upward contraction squeezes stale air out of the lungs from the bottom, helping to expel it more fully. Natural abdominal breathing causes the belly to expand on the in-breath and contract on the out-breath—the breathing of babies.

In reverse abdominal breathing, the in-breath can be through the nose or the

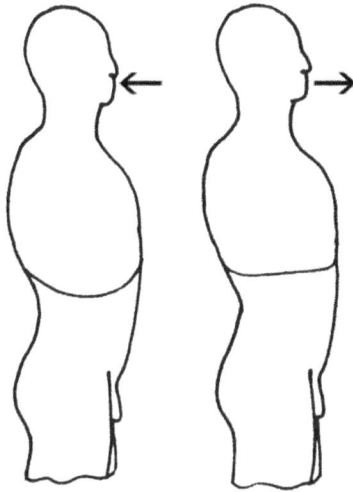

Figure 4.2 Natural abdominal breathing causes the diaphragm to pull down evenly on the in-breath and push up on the out-breath.

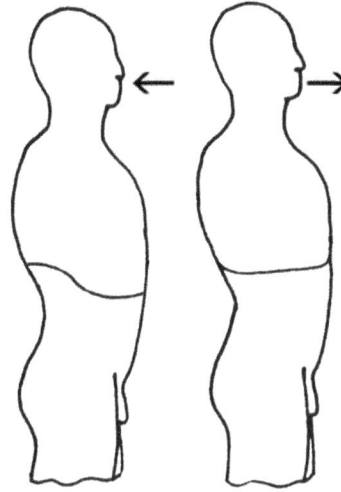

Figure 4.3 Reverse abdominal breathing causes the back part of the diaphragm to rise and the front part to pull down on the in-breath.

mouth, and the out-breath is through the nose. The practice consists of contracting the back half of the diaphragm upward and backward and expanding the front half of the diaphragm downward, which pulls the bottom of the lungs downward and to the front for the in-breath. (Figure 4.3) Then the front half of the diaphragm contracts upward and the back half relaxes downward for the out-breath, again flattening the diaphragm. Reverse abdominal breathing causes the belly to contract on the in-breath and expand on the out-breath—the reverse of natural abdominal breathing.

Natural abdominal breathing, as its name implies, is an innate way to breath—again, witness the breathing of infants and very young children. Reverse abdominal breathing, on the other hand, is a learned—and, ultimately, forced—process. There is a great deal of controversy regarding the efficacy and safety of reverse breathing. Proponents recommend it because it amps-up the chi rather quickly, imparting greater power in a shorter span of time. Detractors say that because it is a forced and artificial method, it can lead to high blood pressure, acid reflux, hemorrhoids, and even insanity.

I cannot personally vouch for the stances of either the proponents or the detrac-

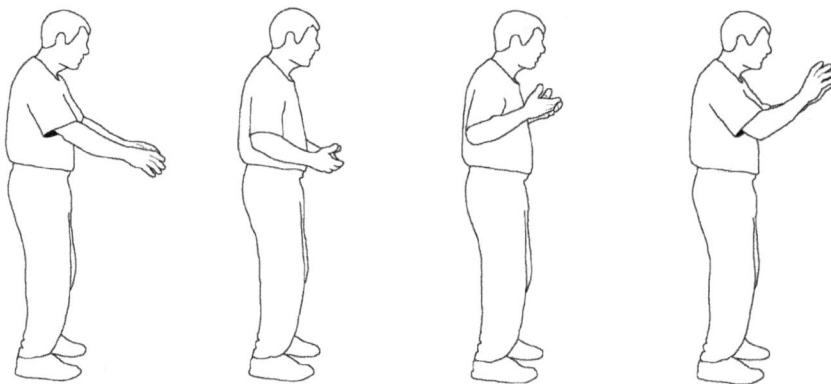

**Figure 4.4** In the Heng and Hah breathing exercise, as you breathe in deeply and gather energy, say, "Heng" (left three images), and as you breathe out sharply, say, "Hah!" (right).

## Heng and Hah

I first heard of the abdominal breathing exercise knowns as "Heng and Hah" as a way to strengthen reverse abdominal breathing, but I've found it effective with natural abdominal breathing, too. However, unlike the breathing of natural abdominal breathing, which goes in and out silently through the nose, the breathing of Heng and Hah is all through the mouth and is accompanied by a vocalization. To perform this exercise, you breathe in with a deep natural abdominal in-breath while vocalizing the word "Heng," then you breathe out by contracting the abdominal muscles while vocalizing the word "Hah." The vocalizations can be explosive, but need not be for general practice. To enhance the experience, you can perform a movement reminiscent of Push, where the hands scoop in toward the belly and rise toward the chest on the Heng, then push outward at chest level on the Hah. The more explosive the out-breath, the more sharply you should jolt the arms outward. This exercise not only deliberately deepens the breath, it exercises the abdominal muscles and links the abdominal breathing process, in and out, to a pulling in of energy then an expulsion of it. (Figure 4.4)

tors because, while I sometimes practice reverse breathing, my personal preference is natural breathing—precisely because it is natural. And it strikes me that reverse breathing is, in addition, totally unnecessary and may actually—over a length of time—produce weaker results. My research, as reflected in *The Wellspring*, indicates that it is not the air of breathing, per se, that generates the chi in the abdomen and then drives it through the chi system, but the rhythmic, mechanical, downward pressure of the lungs and diaphragm on the viscera. If this is the case, then natural breathing is preferable because it causes the lungs and diaphragm to press downward more thoroughly and as a single unit against the viscera.

However, reverse breathing helps create the chi ball in the belly—the tantien—and with practice, one can learn to roll this ball in various ways. The sensations of this can be quite strong as you learn to link the rolling sensation with the breath, external movement, and chi to more powerfully propel the gestalt of these forces and energies through the cycles and curves of the tai chi symbol. This is why fa jin can sometimes be more potent when propelled by reverse breathing.

But even if reverse breathing can make the chi flow more strongly, that doesn't mean it flows more powerfully, in and of itself, although its speed might make it seem to. Power comes not just from speed or directional guidance, but from the sheer quantity of chi flowing through the meridians, and for that to occur, the meridian system must be opened completely. It is my personal belief that natural breathing and reverse breathing are the yin and yang of breathing. Natural breathing is the yin, gently opening the meridians with progressively increasing chi pressure that is pushed gently when performing the form, but rapidly when utilizing Tai Chi martially. Reverse breathing is the yang of breathing, adding two elements: suddenly increased chi to power the movements and rotation of the chi ball in the tantien to accomplish directional movements. I'll discuss this chi ball shortly.

That sudden increase in power is exactly why some practitioners believe that reverse breathing, if practiced to the exclusion of natural breathing, might indeed have negative physiological repercussions. As anyone who exercises knows, you can't just start out full bore. You must work into any routine or risk injury. Such a situation is bad enough when dealing with external exercises, the overdoing of which can lead to strained muscles, stressed or torn tendons and ligaments, and other injuries. But when dealing with internal energy work, the dangers are potentially more serious. Just as one must gradually strengthen muscles and tendons when doing external exercises, one should gradually strengthen and open the meridian system—the channels that carry chi flow—before attempting to pump higher loads of chi through it.

I'll go into the meridian system later, but for now, it's important to realize that gradual development of it includes not simply generating a more powerful chi flow, but loosening and eliminating blockages that prevent chi from circulating freely throughout the body. It avails little to try to pump strong flows through weak channels or channels that are tied up here and there with blockages. To do so would only invite, at best, disruption, and at worst, backups of chi that could lead to serious and permanent harm. Tai Chi is a very natural and gradual way to develop mastery over oneself at all levels, and I believe that natural breathing is more in tune, in its methods, with that goal for the average practitioner who is

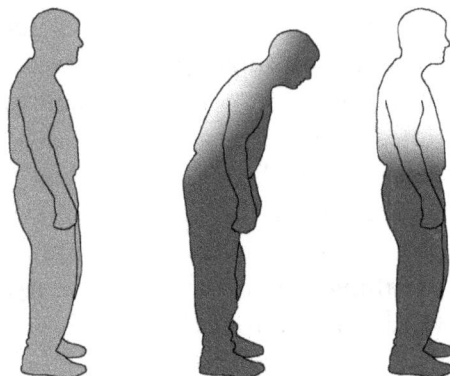

Figure 4.5 A diffuse chi body fills the body (left). A bent body condenses the chi body improperly (center). Correct body alignments allow the chi body to condense into the legs and lower torso (right).

seeking health and self-development. The more serious practitioner might indulge in reverse breathing, and the martially inclined should definitely practice it but also should seek to achieve a balance between increasing power and providing the means to adequately express it.

We remember from the Tai Chi Classics that "the mind motivates the chi, and the chi then motivates the body." I've asked many people about how it feels inside when they are startled, say, by a loud and sudden noise. Most agree that it feels as if something inside them—a sort of shadow body—jumps, then the physical body follows, as if elastically snapped back into alignment with the shadow body, producing the abrupt jolt the body makes. The shadow body is the chi body. In a very real sense, the Tai Chi practitioner tries to use his art to consciously sense this chi body, strengthen it, control it, and manipulate it at will, all of which cause the practitioner to work toward total body awareness and control.

The chi body is affected by the alignments of the physical body. This is why it is important to maintain a generally upright posture. Try this experiment: Stand with your feet parallel and about shoulder-width apart, then lean forward from your waist and sense what it feels like inside your upper torso and head. You will feel as if your chest grows heavy, your shoulders become tighter, and your head fills with

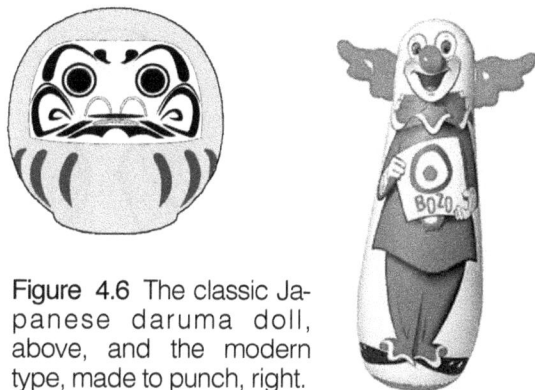

Figure 4.6 The classic Japanese daruma doll, above, and the modern type, made to punch, right.

pressure. Then gradually settle back and straighten. If you are relaxed—not limp—when you straighten, the sensations of heaviness, tension, and pressure will begin to drain downward into your lower torso. (Figure 4.5)

Think of the chi body as if it is water vapor that assumes the same shape as your body. When you bend over at the waist, the bend traps some of the vapor in the upper torso, causing it to remain diffusely there, creating the feeling of pressure inside the head. But straightening the torso allows all of the vapor to condense and drain out of the upper body and settle into the lower torso and legs. This is reflected in the maxim from the Tai Chi Classics: "Heavy on bottom, light on top." Tai Chi has been likened to the daruma doll and those punching-bag dolls that are weighted on the bottom but hollow on the top so that if they are pushed over, they simply roll back upright. (Figure 4.6)

The type of breathing one uses significantly affects not only what happens to this chi body, but where a person's self-awareness is located. If one uses chest breathing, then one's chi—and therefore, self-awareness—remains floating in the chest, and each breath pushes the chi upward from there and into the head. This is why the emotion of anger surges from the chest into the head, why emotionally upset people are, quite literally, unstable, and why flushing, panting, and mental confusion go hand-in-hand with anger, excitement, and panic.

Furthermore, in the average person, chi floating in the chest creates a separation between the upper and lower portions of the body, causing the individual to be disconnected from his foundation. The situation is much like attempting to stand a pyramid on its point rather than on its base. An experienced martial artist can easily take advantage of this sort of imbalance to topple an opponent, but in everyday life, the imbalance causes the individual to be unstable on his feet. Younger people can compensate for this instability by using other muscles inappropriately to help stabilize the body, but as people grow older and their musculature atrophies and becomes less responsive, there is less and less external muscular support. Hence, falling from overbalance is quite common among the elderly.

I remember reading many years ago a report on a survey in which criminologists asked muggers how they chose their victims. The consensus was that the critical factors were not just place and circumstance—isolated areas where the mugger could act without witnesses or interference—but also how the potential victims carried themselves. Muggers tend to victimize those who not only seem less aware of their surroundings but also whose tread is unstable. The victims are seen, quite literally, as pushovers.

Abdominal breathing, on the other hand, in conjunction with proper alignment, relaxation, and other factors, trains one, over time, to sink the chi body into the lower part of the body, or metaphorically, to the tantien. This has several effects, all positive. First, it assists in promoting inner calm. Second, it sinks the center of bodily self-awareness into the lower half of the body rather than pushing it upward into the chest and head, giving the individual greater emotional, as well as physical, stability. And when the chi—or the chi body—sinks into the lower abdomen and legs, it compacts, becoming denser and more powerful, particularly in the region of the tantien. Some Tai Chi exponents refer to this increased density as "the filling." I call it the "chi belly." For those who value a flat stomach, this has the unfortunate effect of giving you a slight (or sometime not-so-slight!) pot belly. As you become more aware of this greater density, you also will be-

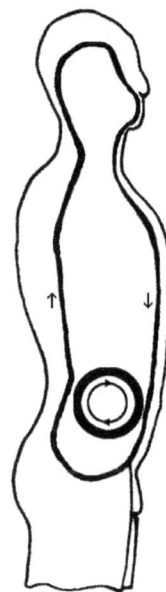

Figure 4.7 When the chi is sunken into the tantien, it is possible to rotate the central portion of it to further increase the chi's production and flow.

come aware that at its core you can use reverse breathing, as discussed earlier, to create an energized rolling ball of chi whose rotation is tied to the abdominal breathing process. With each rotation, the ball drives chi into through the body in different ways according to the direction the ball is rolled. (Figure 4.7)

Whatever you chose to call the chi belly, the important factor is that the preponderance of the chi is now located below the lungs rather than hovering around them. So, when you apply abdominal breathing, the physical action of breathing pushes downward in a muscular wave onto and through the viscera, the physiological and symbolic center of which is the tantien, where the chi is generated. This not only amplifies the chi but gives it greater impetus through the entire chi system and further helps settle one's awareness into the lower portions of the body. Again, see *The Wellspring* for a fuller description of the mechanism of chi generation and movement, but in essence, the surge of chi up the spine happens because, when the abdomen contracts on an abdominal out-breath, the chi that is in the viscera in a relatively diffuse state is suddenly compressed from above and pushed into the channel of the spine, which is not only extremely conductive of chi energy but also is of a narrower diameter, which amps-up the pressure. Think of water flowing through a hose being constricted and given greater power by a nozzle. This is why the back and spine are yang and "light up" with energy and is part of the reason the Tai Chi Classics say that "the chi adheres to the back."

There is one final note to make on breathing. In general, and except for specific instances in some chi kung forms, all breathing should be in and out through the nose. Breathing in through the nose is more conducive to deep, relaxed breathing, and it causes the air to flow more deeply into the lungs. Breathing in through the mouth, on the other hand, tends to localize the in-breath in the chest, which defeats the purpose of abdominal breathing in general.

The ancient practitioners of chi kung...deduced ways to control and regulate the seemingly automatic breathing function, which they saw as voluntary. By deliberately controlling the breathing process, they found that other functions of the body—heartbeat, blood flow, and many other physical and emotional functions—could be consciously altered. The mind, said chi kung practitioners, can control and manipulate the flow of energy that is created through proper breathing. Therefore the mind, coordinated with breathing, can be responsible for the state of one's physical health, one's blood pressure, one's immune system, and one's mental condition. A chi kung expert can channel the inner energy to any location in the body at will. In other words, the accomplished practitioner can "think" this inner energy to any destination in the body where it is needed.

—Nancy Zi[23]

Symbolically, to breathe is to assimilate spiritual power. Yoga exercises place particular emphasis upon breathing, since it enables man to absorb not only air but also the light of the sun. Concerning solar light, the alchemists had this to say: "It is a fiery substance, a continuous emanation of solar corpuscles which, owing to the movement of the sun and the astral bodies, is in a perpetual stare of flux and change, filling all the universe.... We breathe this astral gold continuously." The two movements—positive and negative—of breathing are connected with the circulation of the blood and with the important symbolic paths of involution and evolution. Difficulty in breathing may therefore symbolize difficulty in assimilating the principles of the spirit and of the cosmos. The "proper rhythm" of Yoga-breathing is associated with the "proper voice" demanded by the Egyptians for the ritual reading of the sacred texts. Both are founded upon imitation of the rhythms of the universe.

—J. E. Cirlot[24]

# ⑤ The Tai Chi Bow

In the midst of his perplexity, he is unaware that my bow already has a drawn arrow which is about to fly. At this moment, I am like the bow, and my opponent becomes the arrow. The energy. is release so fast that the opponent is thrown with the speed of an arrow.

—Yang Cheng-fu[25]

**Tai Chi produces** an elastic power that can rapidly inflate like an airbag, strike out with a whipping action, or create a sudden pull. Also it often is likened to drawing a bow and releasing an arrow. One of my Tai Chi compatriots, Sifu Ray Abeyta, commented to me, "The bow is here," indicating the lumbar vertebrae of his back. I'd been thinking about the bow concept, and his comment made sense, but I respectfully think that the lumbar vertebrae, while crucial, are not the whole of the story.

Let's look first at what it means to use the bow metaphor in relation to Tai Chi. The power of a bow lies in the elasticity of it's limbs. When the archer nocks an arrow then draws the string, the limbs of the bow flex, storing energy. When the archer releases the string, the stored energy whips the limbs back into their original shape, snapping the bowstring against the butt of the arrow, sending it flying. Most Tai Chi movements embody a similar elastic storage and release, although it is more

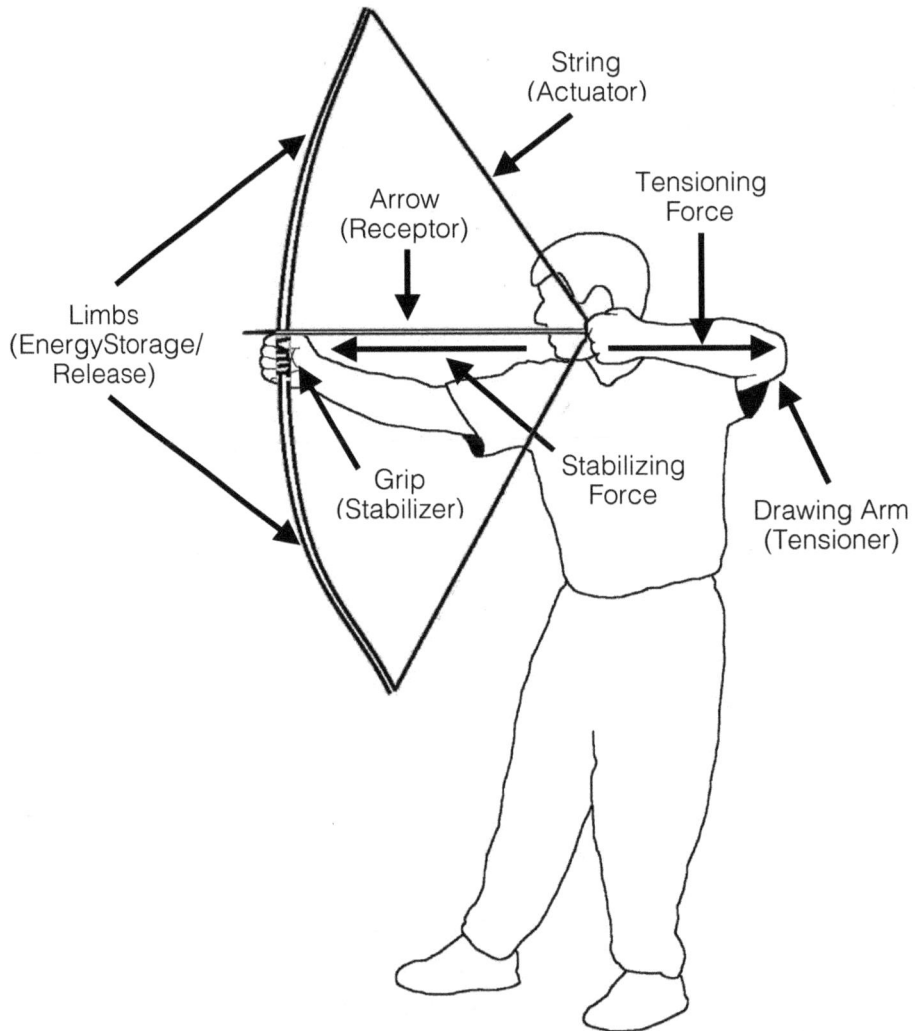

Figure 5.1 The elements of a bow.

apparent in some movements than in others. But before we look at a specific example, we have to take a look at the bow itself to define the parameters of "bowness."

Five elements comprise a bow's energy storage/release system: the bow limbs, the grip, the string, the arm that draws the string, and the arrow. (Figure 5.1) The limbs are the specific sites of energy storage/release—it is the flexibility of their bending then whipping back into their original shape that gives the bow its power. When the limbs are apart, they embody a passive yin state, and when they are drawn together, they embody an energetic yang state that, upon release, swiftly returns to the passive yin state as well as to the limbs' greatest opposition.

But to be stored and released in a bow, the energy must first have a mechanism to activate the storage and release. This is the string—the actuator. The string is, essentially, the physical ability of the system to purposefully manipulate the yin and yang aspects of the bow.

As we all know, however, if you just pick up a bow by the string, the string will not bend the limbs because, as physics tells us, for every force, there must be an equal and opposite force. In the case of the bow, the inward force that pulls backward on the string is exactly balanced by the outward force of the arm and hand that hold the bow steady. Thus, the bow's grip is the point around which the energy storage/release system stabilizes so that it can actually store energy and release it properly. In addition, the grip is the solid connection between the two limbs of the bow that unites the limbs' yin and yang aspects and enables them to work together to perform the task of firing the arrow.

The grip, in turn, is energetically opposite to the tensioning force. This tensioning force is what invests energy into the system. In an archer's bow, the tensioner is the physical act of using arm muscles to draw back the bowstring, transferring energy from the archer into the bow's limbs.

And finally, there must be a mechanism through which the released energy is transformed into a real-world application. This is the arrow—the receptor. The arrow lies exactly along the line of the opposing yin/yang forces of the stabilizing and tensioning forces, which, physically, is at right angles to the actuating string and the storage/release mechanism of the limbs bending inward. This reminds me of the fact that, during Chan-ssu Chin, the plane of the receptor vertical tai chi symbol described by the arm is at right angles to the plane of the actuating horizontal tai chi symbol described by the waist and hip movement.

To summarize: The energy storage/release system of a bow consists of an energy storage/release mechanism (the two limbs), a stabilizer (the grip), an actuator (the string), a tensioner (the energy of the arm drawing the string back), and a receptor (the arrow). The bow has one very solid yin spot—the grip—and one very energetic yang spot—the point on the string where the tensioning hand draws it back. These two spots are at opposite ends of the receptor/arrow, and during the drawing of the bow, both of them increase the amplitude of their state: As the yang force pulls back the string, increasing its energy potential, the yin force of the grip must grow equally firm in balance. At the same time, the bow limbs, which bend inward toward each other on a plane perpendicular to the line of the tensioner/grip polarity, go from a relaxed yin state to a dynamic yang state. Described another way, in a sense, when one draws and releases a bow, the whole system goes from the state of wu chi—a primordial state without action—to the state of tai chi—a state where forces differentiate into yin and yang and become active before reverting back to wu chi again.

All of these elements of the bow have analogs in many, if not most, Tai Chi movements. I'll begin with the stabilizer: the grip. In an actual bow, the grip is stabilized by the archer's forward arm, but in Tai Chi movements the stabilizing element is not an arm but one leg or the other. One leg or the other must be the stabilizing force holding the Tai Chi bow's grip because the body, under the circumstances of normal reality, can stabilize only against the Earth. In Tai Chi parlance, the stabilizer is the yin, or weighted and relatively inactive leg. In a Bow Stance, it is the forward leg; in a Sitting Stance, it is the back leg. Whichever leg it is, that leg's main connection with the body is at the hip, and the main transference point where that leg stabilizes and balances the upper body is in the lumbar region—the first group of vertebrae above the pelvic structure. In other words, the supporting leg functions as the arm the Tai Chi "archer" uses to hold the bow's grip, which is the lumbar vertebrae. In this respect, I agree with Ray that the lumbar vertebrae are vital to the Tai Chi bow because they are the grip around which the forces of the two storage/release limbs are manipulated and a principal point where one must concentrate one's attention.

This leaves the nonsupporting leg, the two arms, and the torso (which includes the head). Any two working together can serve as the Tai Chi bow's limbs, though usually the Tai Chi bow's limbs are the yang (active, nonsupporting) leg and the torso from lumbar to crown point of the head. Usually, one of the chuanist's arms functions as the tensioner (the arm pulling the string back), and the other arm is the receptor (arrow).

The operation of the actuator is a bit more esoteric. As any seasoned Tai Chi practitioner knows, it is not musculature, per se, that creates jin force. In fact, tensed or hardened muscles actually inhibit the flow of chi and the expression of jin. But how is one supposed to use as little muscular force as possible and yet still be able to move the body through the various postures of the Tai Chi form and then release large amounts of energy? Recall the maxim from the Tai Chi Classics: "Heavy on bottom, light on top." This points to the reality that one does use considerable muscular contraction and release to execute the Tai Chi movements, but almost all of that muscular effort takes place in the waist, hips, legs, and feet—the portion of the body lying below the tantien. The upper body should feel loose and empty of muscular effort—not limp, but relaxed and elastically connected to the lower body.

So, how can one move relaxed limbs without muscular effort? Some would say that such an act is impossible, but let's look at three ways to, say, lift your arm above your head: You could use muscles to lift it, but that puts tension in the arm and does not connect the movement of the arm to whole-body movement. You can swing an arm back and forth, using alternate pumping of the legs, until it arcs up and over your head, and while this does entail whole-body movement, the result might be limp, mechanical, and mindless rather than relaxed, flexible, and purposeful. Or you can use what Tai Chi uses: the sinews—predominantly, the fasciae.

The sinews are tough bands of fibrous connective tissue made of collagen that are capable of withstanding and holding elastic tension. There are three types: Ligaments join bone to bone to hold joints together, tendons join muscle to bone to enable transfer of movement from muscle to bone, and fasciae connect muscles to other muscles.[26] The fasciae exist in shorter segments to connect and coordinate the movement of localized muscle groups—say, the various muscles of the calf—and in longer "trains" to link major muscle groups together for movements that engage multiple body parts, such as the entire leg. Figure 5.2 depicts most of the major fascial trains.

Through constant practice, the Tai Chi exponent learns to eliminate gross muscular movement above the waist and to move the upper body, as much as possible, using the contraction and release of the fasciae and tendons. This is another good reason for the slowness of Tai Chi practice. Moving rapidly, which in the untrained person entails only muscular activity, would make it practically impossible for the novice to learn to loosen the muscles yet still move. Slow movement gives the practitioner an opportunity to relax the muscles while learning to move the torso and limbs using the contraction and expansion of fasciae and tendons rather than contraction of muscles. In reality, however—say in practical use for self-defense applications—the exponent does engage some of the muscles of the upper body but does so in appropriate ways that build off the contraction and release of the fasciae and tendons rather than impede their movements through tenseness. Constantly stretching and contracting the

Superficial Back Line                                                 Arm Lines

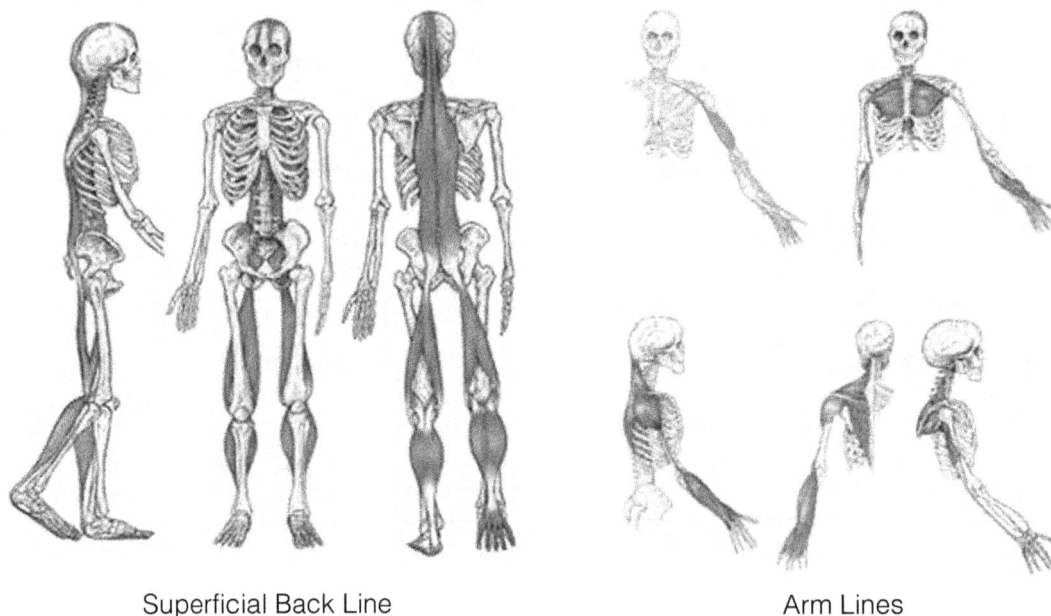

**Figure 5.2** Most of the major fascial trains: The superficial back line corresponds to the two limbs of the most-often used Tai Chi bow. (Shown from the side, front, and back.) Notice how this fascial line arcs over the top of the skull and anchors above the eye sockets. Other fascial trains facilitate other particular Tai Chi bow movements. The spiral line (shown here on only one side) has an obvious correlation to Tai Chi's twisting and torquing. And notice how it, along with the deep and superficial front lines, spirals around the leg, just as chi energy spirals down and up the leg then through the torso to help create fa jin. The arm lines correspond to the same areas through which chi flows down/outward along the inside of the arms and up/inward along their outsides. The lateral line helps in creating alignments along the three vertical axes.[27]

fasciae and tendons is what helps impart greater and continuing flexible power to the Tai Chi player over time, while in the untrained person, these structures lose their elasticity, inhibiting movement and increasing stiffness with age.

The contraction and release of the elastic fasciae (for larger movements) and tendons (for smaller movements) is, I believe, the principal physiological component of the physical force produced by the internal martial arts, while the contraction and release of muscles is the principal component of the physical strength produced by the external martial arts. (Both also employ the more esoteric chi energy, though in different ways. Here, though, I'm dealing strictly with physical move-

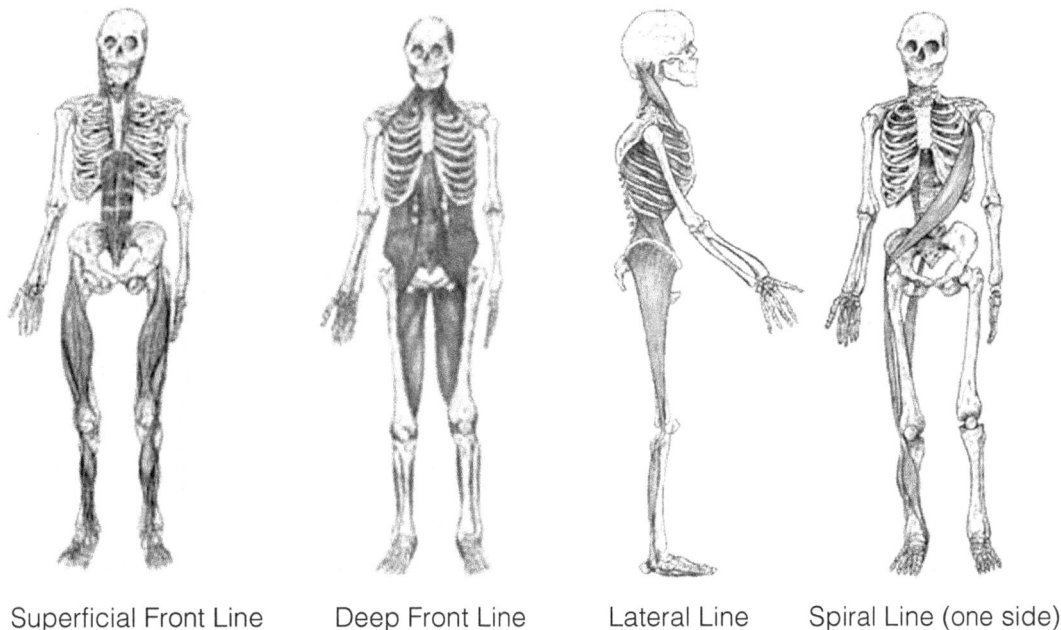

Superficial Front Line    Deep Front Line    Lateral Line    Spiral Line (one side)

ment. I'll discuss chi and its functions in the next chapter.) So, when I refer to "tension" in the descriptions below, it is not muscular tension (hardness), which should be avoided because it not only cramps the flow of chi but also blocks sensitivity to its flow and inhibits the loose movements necessary to manipulate the fasciae and tendons to create the twisting and whipping movements that are characteristic of Tai Chi. Instead, it is a tension that is more akin to treating your fasciae and tendons like elastic bands that can be consciously compressed, stretched, or twisted and then released, causing them to snap back into their original shape.

The superficial back fascial line, in particular, is vitally important for the Tai Chi bow. Figure 5.2 makes it abundantly clear that this fascia comprises the two limbs of the major Tai Chi bow—at least for most Tai Chi movements. Other fasciae come into play for extending and contracting the limbs, twisting, turning, and other movements.[28] The spiral, deep front, and superficial front lines, for example, are critical to twisting, lateral, and cross-body movements like Cloudy Hands and Ward Off, and the various arm lines interact with the spiral line and superficial back line to transmit force through the arms. In fact, any version of the Tai Chi bow is going to use multiple fascial trains, though the specific combination of trains used will vary with the exact composition of the bow, which relates to function and purpose.

I'll leave most of these combinations to the reader's imagination and experimentation, but I'll look at these ideas with regard to Split, though I think they can be applied to most, if not all, Tai Chi movements. I'll use Split as represented by Slant Flying, which is common to most Tai Chi styles and which clearly demonstrates the Tai Chi bow. To perform Slant Flying, the player pushes off of one leg (the yang leg), onto the opposite leg (yin leg), and draws back the arm and hand that are on the same side as the pushing leg along the upper circumference of a flattened Ward Off oval. At the same time, he uses the underside of the flattened Ward Off oval to extend the arm that is on the same side as the stabilizing leg. (Figure 5.3)

One can perform this movement without any internal force—without contracting and releasing the superficial back line—but the resulting movement is empty of energy and would have to rely on muscular strength to produce a reaction and wouldn't be very bow-like. Or one can, through this movement, create a pulling sensation that contracts the superficial back and arm lines, storing an extremely elastic energy in the two limbs of the Tai Chi bow: the pushing leg (from lumbar to heel) and the torso (lumbar to crown of the head). As the pushing leg transfers the body weight to the supporting leg, the segments of the superficial back line inside the pushing leg and torso begin to feel as if they are drawn together by an elastic connection and become more and more dense with compressed energy.

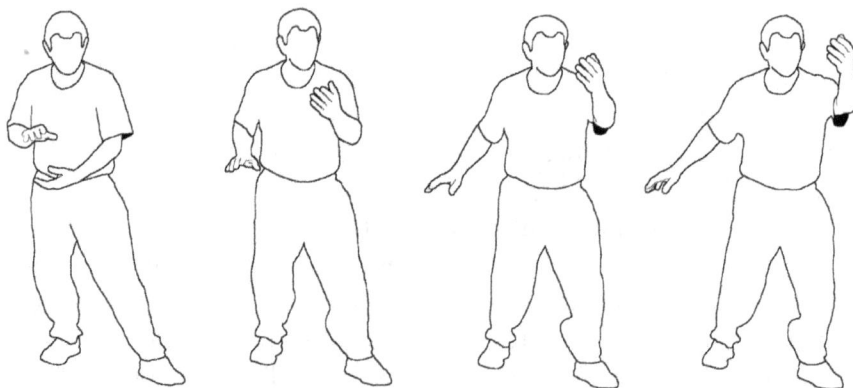

Figure 5.3 The Tai Chi bow illustrated in the movement Slant Flying: no tension in the bow (left), drawing the tension along the superficial back fascial and arm lines with the right hand (center two), and releasing the tension with the right hand, sending the left arm flying (right).

The tensioner that performs the drawing action is the arm and hand that are on the same side as the yang leg. This happens because the exponent has trained his or her body to link other fascial trains, especially those of the arm and shoulder, to the superficial back line and pull it into contraction. This linkage between the fascial trains is the actuator (string). In fact, the exponent is trained through performing the Tai Chi form to consciously (or, at higher levels, instinctively) engage different fascial groups with the superficial back line in various ways. This mental process is often referred to as "mind intent." In other words, one mentally causes particular fascial groups to engage with each other—particularly with the superficial back line—and uses that connection of fascial trains to pull tension into the Tai Chi bow's limbs.

As the tensioning arm, linking and pulling on the appropriate fascial trains, moves in a direction opposite that of the receptor (arrow), which is the other, extended arm, it fills both of the bow limbs with contracted elastic energy. In contrast, both the stabilizing leg and the receptor arm over it feel empty of energy, though in different ways. The supporting leg has the sensation of carrying the weight of the body, but its energy is passive in the sense that the muscles and tendons are relatively inactive outside of their supportive role. The receptor arm over the supporting leg, however, feels empty, just as an arrow seems to be completely empty of energy while a bow is being drawn, even though the drawing action creates a line of potential energy along the shaft of the arrow.

When the elastic tension between the torso and leg that comprise the bow's limbs is suddenly released—again, a mental act of releasing the elastic compression of the fasciae of the drawing arm and leg and their connections to the superficial back line to allow the superficial back line to snap back into its relaxed yin state—the arrow shaft of potential energy abruptly becomes completely kinetic as it absorbs the energy released by the bow limbs. This transfers the energy through the physical structure of the arrow arm, sending the arm flying with all the released force. This flying is not wild but is highly controlled, directed, and focused by training the body through performance of the Tai Chi form to release the energy sequentially into the arm through the Nine-Channel Pearl and to remain in a solid, sunken stance on the yin leg. This bow-like release of force and energy is one type of fa jin.

Following the release of an archer's arrow, there is a brief quivering of the bow limbs as they resume their former, non-energetic state, and this is mirrored in the Tai Chi practitioner when his bow limbs—usually the pushing leg and the torso—shake for a moment after the release. There is a general Tai Chi instruction to let the energy of release simultaneously shoot down to the sole of the pushing leg, which bounces against the ground, and rise to the crown of the head. Some practitioners describe the latter as a sensation of the crown point sort of "popping." This popping at the tip of the upper bow limb that counterbalances the bouncing of the foot of the pushing leg is produced by the superficial back line gripping and releasing the top of the skull as the bow contracts and releases.

The contraction and release of the Tai Chi bow can happen only if the body is properly aligned, as indicated by the general Tai Chi instruction to the practitioner to "tuck in the buttocks," which has the twofold effect of causing the coccyx to point downward and straightening the lumbar vertebrae, and another instruction to "tuck in the chin" to straighten the cervical vertebrae and protrude the inion—the bump at the base of the skull. Failing to comply with these instructions renders the Tai Chi bow useless for the same reasons that disjunctions in the limbs of a real bow would cause the bow to fail to operate. Not straightening the lumbar vertebrae is similar to installing a hinge between the bow's grip and its upper limb. Even if the hinge is situated in such a way that the bow can be drawn, as soon as the energy is released, the bow's upper limb will flop at the grip, the energy will be only weakly transmitted—if at all—from the bow to the arrow, and the arrow will not fly properly. Worse, the energy released by the leg, instead of being controlled at the lumbar grip and directed upward through the torso to the crown, is thrust forward into the belly. (Figure 5.4) This can potentially strain the lumbar vertebrae, and it will certainly fail to accomplish the task of making the arrow fly. Not straightening the cervical vertebrae causes a similar break in the Tai Chi bow's upper limb, terminating the energy not at the tip (crown) but at the base of the neck. (Also Figure 5.4) The result of this can be disastrous because if the energy of the motion is strong enough, the force terminating in and through the neck can cause whiplash.

Another way to look at the dynamics of the Tai Chi bow is to reduce the elements to three: weight, counterweight, pivot point. To illustrate with Wild Horse Tosses Mane: The axis of the supporting leg is the pivot point, the receptor arm—the arm on the weighted side—is the weight (although it only has weight when it is delivering energy), and the actuator arm—the arm on the unweighted side—is the counterweight (which only has weight prior to delivering the energy). The faster and more powerfully you pull back and release the counterweight using elastic energy produced by the fasciae and tendons, the more forcefully the reaction whirls around the pivot point to fill the receptor arm with weight.

There is an interesting double-weighting dynamic at play in Tai Chi bow. This relates to aim, which is important in both archery and Tai Chi. An archer

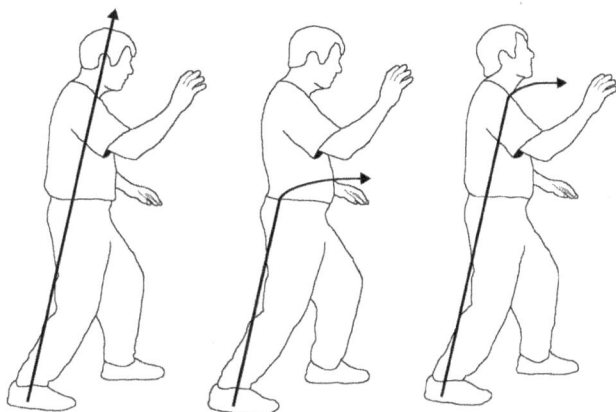

Figure 5.4 The lumbar and cervical vertebrae must be straightened for the Tai Chi bow to function properly. If the bow is formed correctly (left), the energy creates a straight line from the sole to the crown. Failing to straighten the lumbar vertebrae (center) sends the energy out of the front of the belly, while failing to straighten the cervical vertebrae (right) sends it out the front of the neck.

does not pay attention to the arrow as it is drawn but to the target and to the line between the drawing arm and the grip as felt through the string. If these are aligned properly, the arrow will fly true.

In Tai Chi, one also must pay attention to the way the energy of the bow limbs is directed to the target through the line between the tensioner and stabilizer, as felt through the actuating mind intent, to the target, rather than to the receptor arm. If you pay attention to the receptor arm, your attention will cause the force of the energy to stagnate in the arm and make it attempt to apply its own force rather than simply be propelled. What is happening is that one has quit using the fascial structure of the drawing arm to contract and release the superficial back line, and is instead attempting to use the muscles of the receptor arm inappropriately to do the work. It would be like an archer trying to push the arrow forward with muscular strength instead of making it fly through release of elastic tension.

Putting attention (mind intent) into the limb that functions as the arrow causes the limb to become full of muscular force and stiff when it should be empty of force and flexible so that it can fully and efficiently receive the power of the released actuator. This stiffness can be defined as weight because the limb's solidity anchors it in space/time. But as the function of the bow shows, there can be only one anchor in the Tai Chi bow: the lumbar grip braced by the leg that supports the body weight but does not push. Anchoring the arrow with muscular "weight" not only makes it impossible for the arrow to fly to its target, it also creates a situation of double-weighting: weight on the receptor (arrow) and weight on the stabilizer

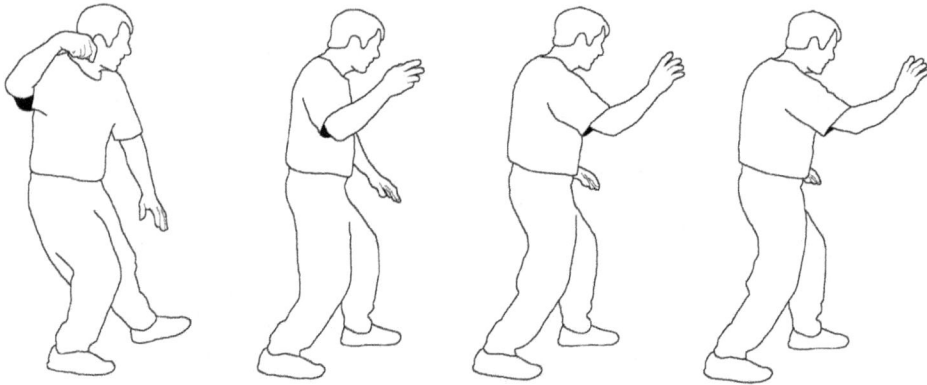

**Figure 5.5** In the Brush Knee Twist Step sequence above, the bow limbs are the torso and right leg, the grip/stabilizer is the left leg, the tensioner is the swinging left arm, the actuator is the composed of the fascial lines connecting the left arm to the superficial back line, and the arrow is the right arm.

(grip). This, in turn, removes mind intent from the drawing of the string, which immediately dissipates the elastic tension on the bow limbs and prevents them from doing their whipping action and causes the movement to be empty of internal force and to emphasize muscular strength.

Ultimately, double-weighting is a fault that operates on various levels to inhibit not just stability, rapid movement, and torquing, but also Tai Chi's flexible expression of power. So the key is to allow all the motions of a given movement to operate freely around a single stabilizer: the weighted leg. The energy from the other, active, leg can then enter the waist and be directed from there through the torso into the receptor, be it into the arm on the same side (Press), into the arm of the opposite side (Ward Off), straight forward/backward (Push), or circularly (Roll Back).

So, in Slant Flying, you don't put energy into the forward arm, which is the receptor. Instead, you concentrate on the tensioner—the arm that is pulling backward and downward with elastic tension—and on the line of force that is subsequently drawn. Then, when you release the energy, it will whip through your body and into the receptor arm. As you release the arrow, your attention should not shift to the arm, or even to your target, but into the distance beyond your target. This helps ensure that your energy is directed fully into and through your target and helps psychologically deemphasize the musculature of the receptor arm by making it seem as if the target is far off, even if it actually is close.

In Split movements, the tensioner arm moves directly away from the receptor arm, but in Press movements, such as Press, Punch, and Brush Knee Twist Step, the tensioner arm is the one that suddenly pulls, pushes, or swings perpendicularly to the receptor arm as discussed in the section on Press. (Figure 5.5) Ward Off movements exhibit a cross-body bow, that uses the spiral lines and deep and superficial front lines as much as they do the superficial back line, such as when Monkey Moving Backward is used as a backwards throw. (Figure 5.6)

The bow concept is very visible in some movements and less so in others, such as the movement Rolling the Ball, whether it is used as a throw against someone grasping your arms, as a foot and ankle twist defense against a front heel or side kick, or for other purposes. Here, the weighted leg is the stabilizer, the non-weighted leg and torso are the bow limbs, the hand rolling downward is the tensioner, and the hand rolling upward is the receptor. (Figure 5.7)

However, I want to stress that there are many notable exceptions to the functions of the various body parts. While the stabilizer/grip must always be the weighted leg because that is what provides your foundation, the bow limbs need not always be the torso and the other leg, the tensioner/drawing force need not always come from one of the arms, and the receptor/arrow need not always be an arm. The receptor can be any part of an arm—elbow, say—a leg, or even the torso. In Shoulder Strike, for example, which can use the upper back or hip as well as the shoulder, the energy does not travel completely through the Nine-Channel Pearl, but terminates either in channel three (hip) or channel four (the shoulder or upper back).

Similarly, in some movements, the roles of the different body parts can interchange. In the odd Wu style movement that follows Golden Cock that we looked at in previous chapters, the stabilizer is the weighted leg, the tensioner is the lower arm, the bow limbs are the torso and the upper arm, and the receptor is the kicking leg. (Figure 5.8) A different configuration is evident in the kicks known as Separate Right Foot and Separate Left Foot. In these, the stabilizer is the weighted leg, the tensioner is the rear, upper arm, the bow limbs are the torso and forward hand, and the receptor is the kicking leg. (Figure 5.9) Kick Forward with the Heel is yet another configuration. Here, the stabilizer is the weighted leg, the receptor is the kicking leg, the bow limbs are both arms, and the tensioner is the torso—the tension created by suddenly sinking the weight of the body. (Figure 5.10)

And finally, some movements are not amenable to defining each individual body part as a discreet bow element, particularly in movements that stress Tai Chi's coiling and uncoiling. In Lotus Swing, for example, where both arms swing togeth-

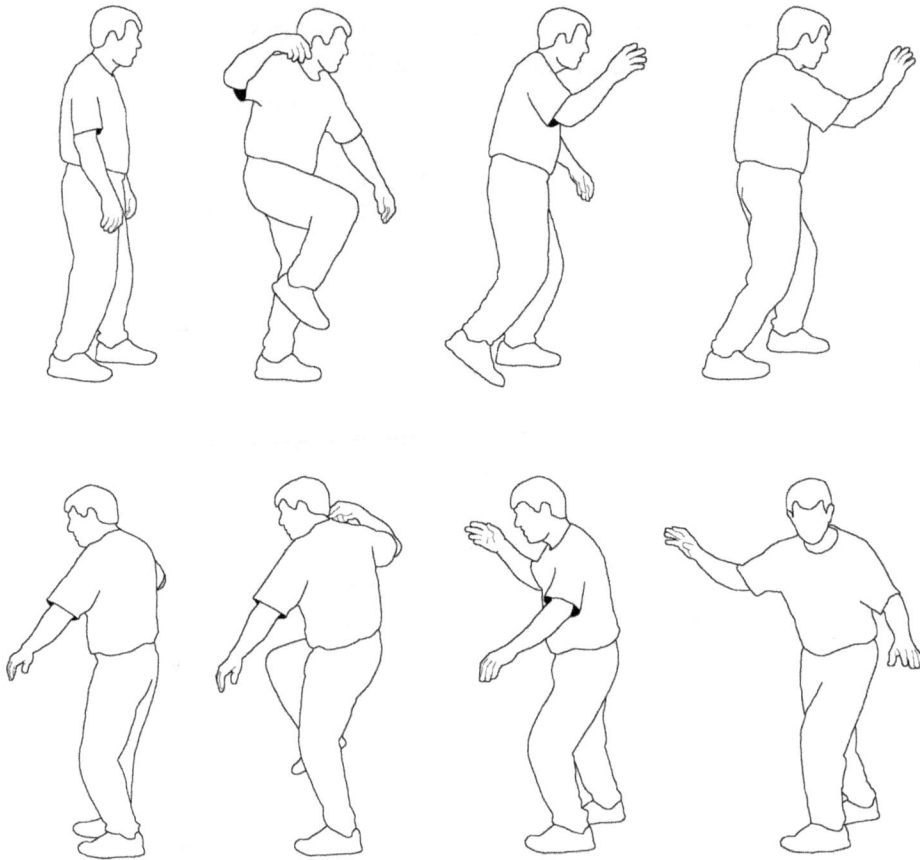

**Figure 5.6** When Monkey Moving Backward is used as a strike or shove, the tensioner is the lower arm (top row), but when it is used as a throw, the tensioner is the the upper arm (bottom row).

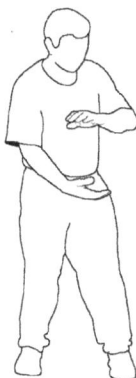

Figure 5.7 Rolling the Ball to twist a foot.

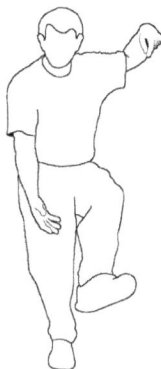

Figure 5.8 The Wu style movement following Golden Cock Stands on One Leg.

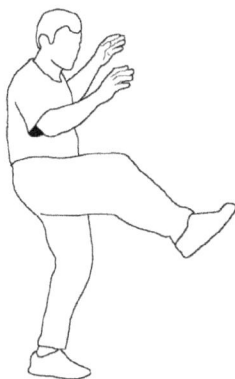

Figure 5.9 Separate Right Foot.

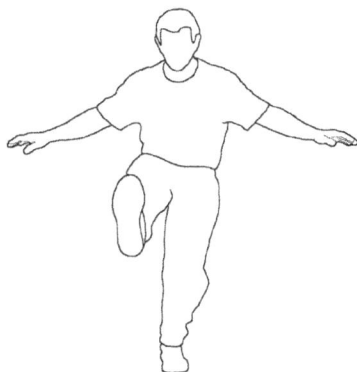

Figure 5.10 Kick Forward with Heel.

er in one direction as the swinging leg arcs up in the opposite direction, it is more useful, perhaps, to think of the weight/counterweight concept.

The arrow, however, in all cases where the bow concept applies, is just the part of the body—usually a limb, but maybe the shoulder, back, or hip—that lies in some straight line of energy perpendicular to the drawing bow string and bending bow limbs. And the bow limbs, while almost always being the torso and, most often, one of the legs, also can be more internalized into, say, the shoulder and hip.

At the very highest levels of achievement, the movements are too small to be perceived outwardly, so perhaps that does locate the entire bow, as Ray Abeyta described, within the lumbar vertebrae. Certainly that is the section of the spine around which the entire action of the bow takes place, and without a solid grip (rooting) there can't be a bow since everything operates around that stabilizing connection to the Earth.

Store up the *chin* (internal strength)
like drawing a bow.

Mobilize the *chin*
like pulling silk from a cocoon.

Release the *chin*
like releasing an arrow.

To *fa chin*,
sink,
relax completely,
and aim in one direction!

In the curved seek the straight,
store,
then release.

—Wu Yu-hsiang[29]

# ⑥ Energy Operations

Speaking of the mechanistic approach of biochemistry, [Albert Szent-Györgyi] pointed out that when experimenters broke living things down into their constituent parts, somewhere along the line life slipped through their fingers and they found themselves working with dead matter. He said, "It looks as if some basic fact about life were still missing, without which any real understanding is impossible." For the missing basic fact, Szent-Györgyi proposed putting electricity back into living things.

—Robert O. Becker[30]

**We'll start this** chapter with a discussion of electricity for reasons that will become obvious as we go along. Electricity is defined as a flow or transfer of electrons or ions from a location of higher energy potential to a location of lower energy potential. The flow or transfer takes place within a conducting medium, which is simply a substance amenable to such a flow or transfer of electrons or ions, such as the copper wire in our familiar household electrical circuits. Metals generally have high conductivity, though there are exceptions, such as lead. There also are many nonmetallic mediums that are efficient conductors of electricity, such as electrolytes, one common example of which is salt water—a substance prevalent in the human body.

In an electrical system, electrical flow through a pair of wires is created by attaching them to the terminals of a power source: a battery or, even better, an electrical generator or dynamo. The other ends of these wires can then be attached to a receiver object, such as a motor, a toaster, or a light bulb, to do work. The electricity flows outward from the electrical source along one wire, through the receiver object, then back to the electrical source through the other wire. When everything is hooked up, the electrical source, wires, and receiver object form a complete circuit. (Figure 6.1) For electricity to flow, there must be a complete, uninterrupted circuit—a switch, for example, can break the circuit so the electricity can't flow if you don't want it to.

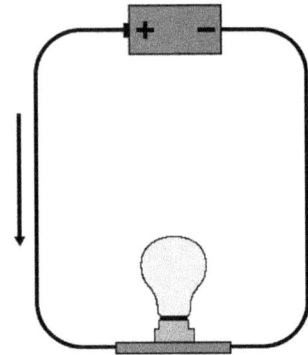

Figure 6.1 A complete electric circuit consists of an unbroken line of electrical energy from the power source to an appliance, and back to the power source.

Two aspects of the flow of electricity through a circuit are important to this discussion: amperage, which is the rate at which the electrical current flows, and voltage, which is the strength with which the current flows. To liken this to water in a pipe— also called the "hydraulic analogy"—amperage is the amount of the water flow—in other words, the amount of water a given pipe can contain. Voltage is the strength of the pressure pushing the water through the pipe. The higher the pressure, the faster—and more powerfully—the water will flow, even though the actual volume of water in the pipe remains the same regardless of pressure.[31]

In a battery, electricity is generated by a chemical reaction, and while a battery has constant electrical potential, its current is comparatively weak. In a generator or its big brother, the dynamo, current flow is created by physically moving magnets rapidly along the axis of a wire. The physical movement of the magnets and wire is effected by an external source, such as the turning of a generator powered by a gasoline engine or the turning of a dynamo powered by water, wind, or steam flowing through a turbine. Generators and dynamos at rest have no electrical potential, but when they are set in motion, they produce an electrical potential that is much more powerful than a battery can generate.

The movement of the magnets along the axis of a wire in a dynamo takes advantage of the link between electricity and magnetism, both of which produce energy fields around the electrical or magnetic object. Magnetic fields moved along the axis of a conducting medium produce an electrical flow in the conductor, and conversely, an electrical flow through a conductor produces a magnetic field—or

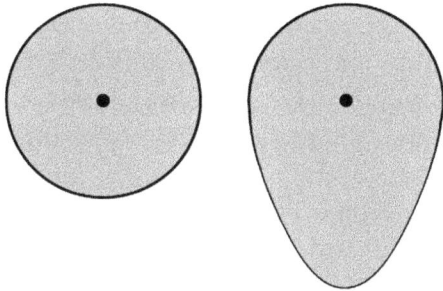

Figure 6.2 In cross section, the electromagnetic field that surrounds an electrical line would be round if there were no gravity (left), but gravity distends the field downward (right).

more properly, an electromagnetic field —around the conductor. Not all electrical fields are electromagnetic because an electromagnetic field is an electrical field in motion. Power plants, which are stationary, produce large electrical fields, and likewise, batteries are surrounded by small electrical fields. But as soon as an electrical current moves through a wire, its field also goes into motion, becoming an electromagnetic field.

Large-scale electrical systems consist of three parts: the power plant, usually a group of dynamos; a switchboard/distribution system, which we usually see as clusters of transformers; and a network of power lines, from large transmission lines that carry electricity to neighborhoods and commercial centers down to smaller wires that permeate the walls of houses and buildings. A power plant is surrounded by a large electrical field. A switchboard/distribution system also is surrounded by an electrical field, but due to the flow of electricity through its various components, this field is shot through with flows and filaments that are electromagnetic in nature. However, because the electromagnetic currents in transformer complexes flow in numerous directions all at once, the cumulative effect on a practical level is an electrical field instead of an electromagnetic flow. And finally, power lines and wires are surrounded only by electromagnetic fields. In the absence of gravity, the electromagnetic fields around wires would be tubular in shape as they run along the length of the wire. But electromagnetic fields are susceptible to gravity, so if one surrounding a wire is looked at in cross section, it would have an egg shape, not a circular one, because gravity pulls downward on it. (Figure 6.2)

Electromagnetism is one of the four fundamental forces of nature, which are "the interactions of physical systems that appear not to be reducible to more basic interactions, and each are understood as the dynamics of a field."[32] The other three fundamental forces are the strong interaction, the weak interaction, and gravitation. The strong interaction, which is responsible for the binding of atomic nuclei, and the weak interaction, which mediates decay in atomic nuclei, both act over minuscule subatomic distances. But gravitation and electromagnetism act upon everyday macroscopic phenomena over potentially infinite distances across the universe. In addition, the electromagnetic force is second in strength only to the strong interaction. It makes sense that the strong interaction would be the strongest of the fundamental forces since it's the one that binds matter together, but this also means that electromagnetism is stronger than gravitation, even if it is affected by it.

Electromagnetic fields, then, can be quite powerful and influential in proximity to their source and can extend infinitely in all directions. But the effects of any field diminishes over distance and eventually becomes indistinguishable from the background noise of the manifold magnetic and electromagnetic fields permeating the substructure of reality. So it's important to note that in the illustrations of fields in this chapter, the boundaries shown do not indicate actual perimeters of the fields but are more to indicate the field's shape and effective range.

When the electromotive force is strong, the current will be abundant, and when the electromotive force is weak, the current will also be feeble. In addition, when the resistance is high, the current will be low, and when the resistance is low, the current will be high, and when the body is tense and stiff, the resistance is high and the current is low.

—Yang Jwing-Ming[33]

# Chi

**The human body**—almost every type of living body for that matter—also generates and conducts electricity. In biological membranes, currents are carried by ionic salts, and the principal conductors are the nerves. *The Wellspring* describes the exact mechanism the body uses to generate this bioelectricity, but in short, physical or chemical stimulation of a nerve causes an energy differential in the nerve, which then produces a flow of ions. And of course, where electricity flows, it is surrounded by an electromagnetic field. My belief is that the bioelectromagnetic fields surrounding the bioelectric flows in the nerves *are* chi. The stimulation that creates the nerves' bioelectrical impulses can come from an outside source tweaking the nerves to create the inbound signals that carry sensory information through the autonomic nervous system to the central nervous system. Stimulation also comes from inside the body. We might think of this stimulation as being a conscious decision to move the body, such as lifting an arm, but while the nerve impulse that impels motion comes from the central nervous system, the majority of the bioelectrical component isn't created there but merely channeled through it. To see where most of the bio-electricity does come from, it's useful to look at the close parallels between the body's nervous system and large-scale electrical systems.

Like large-scale electrical systems, the nervous system of the human body has three main components. The first is the central nervous system, which consists of the brain and spinal cord. The second is the peripheral nervous system, which consists of the somatic nerves, which transmit the impulses that result in voluntary movement, and the autonomic nerves, which take in sensory information and control non-voluntary impulses such as the heartbeat and glandular secretions. Both of these systems are well known to the layman. But there is a third component that is less well known and that, in the past, has been lumped together with the peripheral nervous system. However, research physician Michael D. Gershon has argued convincingly that this component is actually independent of the peripheral nervous system and of equal importance to both it and the central nervous system.[34]

It is the *enteric plexus*, which is a mass of neurons located within the muscular linings of the digestive tract and which Gershon refers to as the "second brain." He calls it that because the enteric plexus contains more neurons than the entire peripheral nervous system and spine taken together; only the brain itself has more neurons. The enteric plexus also operates independently of both the central and peripheral nervous systems. The connections between the enteric plexus and the central nervous system is only one small strand of nerves—the vagus nerves—and even if the vagus nerves are severed, the enteric plexus continues to operate normally. And the location of the greatest amassing of the digestive tract is, of course, the exact location of the tantien—the physiological structure where, according to Tai Chi tradition and Chinese medicine, chi is generated.

As I said above, bioelectricity can be generated in the nerves though external physical stimulation, which sends sensory signals to the central nervous system. Likewise, the nervous system as a whole generates its own, whole-body bioelectrical flow thanks to internal physical stimulation. This occurs in the enteric plexus, not in the central nervous system, which is almost completely encased in the skull and backbone and is thus insulated from physical pressure. The enteric plexus, on the other hand, is constantly being mechanically stimulated in several ways. The first and primary stimulation is through the normal process of digestion, where the stimulation is provided by the physical presence of food bulk inside the digestive tract. The pressure of food bulk instigates what is called the peristaltic reflex, which is the propensity of the muscles in the gut wall to squeeze rhythmically downward, each squeeze caused by a burst of electrical activity in the gut's neurons that sequentially activates the muscles surrounding the intestinal wall. The main purpose of the peristaltic reflex is to transport food bulk through the intestines, but coincidentally, it also creates a perpetual flow of bioelectrical—and thus bioelectromagnetic—energy that ripples downward through the gut along with the squeezing. This rippling energy always occurs in the intestines, sort of like an engine idling, but it revs up when food bulk creates heightened physical stimulation.

A second, though relatively minor form of mechanical stimulation is caused by bending—to pick up something off the floor, to tie a shoelace—which squeezes the gut. And the third form of mechanical stimulation is breathing. As we saw in the chapter on breathing, chest breathing provides almost no direct stimulation to the gut, but abdominal breathing is an entirely different matter. When one breathes abdominally, the rhythmic downward pressure of the diaphragm on the intestines induces a reaction similar, but on a larger scale, to the normal downward pulses of the peristaltic reflex. The two working together generate more powerful bioelectrical pulses—and hence, a greater bioelectromagnetic flow—than does the peristaltic reflex alone.

We can see here also the reason for the injunction not to perform chi-building exercises such as Tai Chi or chi kung too soon before or after eating. Both processes utilize the same intestinal muscles, but each acts on them in a different way and for different purposes. The presence of food bulk inside the digestive tract causes the peristaltic reflex to happen through internal stimulation, while deep abdominal breathing externally squeezes the same tissue. If the intestines are squeezed naturally from the inside because they are distended by food and simultaneously squeezed from the outside with deep abdominal breathing, the two pressures counteract one another. This has the two-fold effect of interfering with the digestive process and interfering with the gut's ability to use the induced activity of abdominal breathing to rev-up the naturally idling peristaltic reflex to generate larger waves of bioelectrical/bioelectromagnetic energy. By the same token, one also should allow those same nerves and muscles to calm from chi-building exercises before filling the digestive tract with food bulk.

Thus, the enteric plexus, located in the tantien, is the body's electrical dynamo, and we can see how chi-building exercises—particularly the act of abdominal breathing—can cause this dynamo to output higher levels of bioelectric/bioelectromagnetic flow. This flow—whether untrained and relatively weak or trained and strong—is then channeled into the base of the spine, where each exhale pushes it up through the spine and into the brain. The central nervous system is the body's electrical switchboard/distribution system, where the main electrical flow from the dynamo is split off and sent to various locations. And the body's electrical lines and wires are the large and small nerves that carry impulses to and from the central nervous system. These impulses are strongest in the major nerve channels, such as the major nerves that run through a limb, and they are weaker in the smaller channels, such as a nerve that goes into a muscle fiber. (It also is possible to generate chi locally, say in a limb, through stimulating local nerves or nerve groups by simple muscular contraction. This is analogous to using a battery instead of a dynamo to generate electricity, but we'll discuss that later. For now, we're talking about the whole-body system.)

Within the body there is a complex of circuitry running contiguously with the nervous system that is composed of two major sets of channels. Traditional Chinese medicine calls these channels "meridians." Note that the meridians are not the nerve tissue itself, nor are they independent, specialized structures, such as tubes. If actual specialized, physiological strands of tissue are involved, they seem to be elements of the sheathing and tissue surrounding the nerves. (Again, refer to *The Wellspring* for more details on this.) But because the body is saturated with the electrolyte salt water, and since chi is a bioelectromagnetic flow, it doesn't need specialized structures but instead simply flows through the tissue surrounding the nerves, just as an electromagnetic field flows through the air—and even through many forms of tangible matter—surrounding a wire. Hence, the meridians are called "channels" rather than being directly identified as some kind of physiological tubes or strands of tissue.

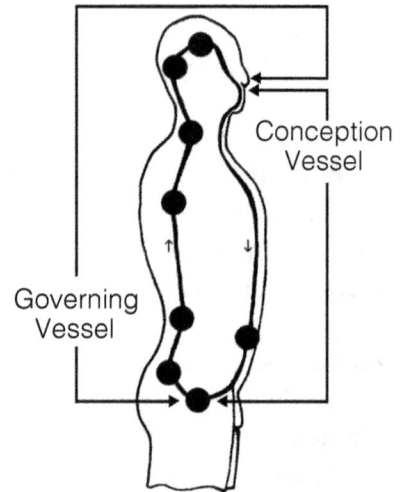

Figure 6.3 The Microcosmic Orbit consists of the body's two primary chi channels: the Conception Vessel and the Governing Vessel.

Traditional Chinese medicine associates strong and continuous flow of chi through the meridians with good health and proper organic functioning. Conversely, blockages that inhibit chi flow can cause or be associated with illness, and injury also causes blockages. Blockages are like breaks or short circuits in electrical lines. As research physician Robert O. Becker has shown, naturally occurring electrical impulses in the body—and, thus, the attendant chi flow—are associated with the innate healing energy of the body. [35] The meridians are what an acupuncturist stimulates with needles to improve the chi flow by using the stimulation to release blockages in the channels to allow the chi to flow more freely or to temporarily increase or block the flow to a particular area of the body. Note that acupuncture needles are made of highly conductive metal, which makes sense if the acupuncturist seeks to affect and influence the bioelectromagnetic flow. Chi flow also can be obstructed by poor posture, tight joints, and tense musculature, much like the flow of water through a garden hose can be constricted by squeezing or kinking the hose, mainly because they kink, compress, or misalign the nerves, inhibiting thorough bioelectric flow. In relation to chi flow, physical misalignments and muscular tension are tantamount to resistance in an electrical circuit, which impede electrical flow.

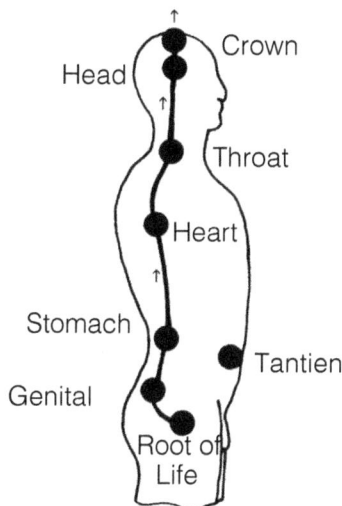

Figure 6.4 The chakras are power centers located on a line contiguous with the Governing Vessel.

The first, and more important, set of channels is the major circuit that generates and distributes the bioelectric/bioelectromagnetic energy. This is called the Microcosmic Orbit, or Small Circulation, and it consists of two primary chi channels: the Conception Vessel and the Governing Vessel. (Figure 6.3) The Conception Vessel, which runs down the front of the body from the tip of the tongue to the tissue between the genitals and anus, called the perineum (the *huiyin* acupuncture point), is primarily composed of the enteric plexus, the generator of chi. The Governing Vessel, which runs from the perineum, up the spine, and through the brain to the hard palate, is the central nervous system, the switchboard/distribution system for chi. Even the names of these two channels identify their functions. The flow of chi through this circuit is ever-present in the living body, and when it ceases, so does life. Many of the body's important energy centers—also called chakras—lie along the Governing Vessel. (Figure 6.4)

In addition to the two primary channels of the Microcosmic Orbit, there are twelve main meridians that branch from specific areas of the Microcosmic Orbit, into the torso and limbs. Each of these twelve main meridians is associated with a principal organ or group of organs, but that is a subject beyond the scope of this book.[36] What concerns us here is that these meridians branch into the limbs: Each limb has three circuits that send chi flowing through each limb. The outward flow, whose meridians are associated with the somatic nerves, sends action signals to the body. The inward flow, whose meridians are associated with the autonomic nerves, conducts sensory input to the brain. Each of these twelve major meridians branch further, along with the nerves, into all of the body's tissues. This is the network of the body's electrical lines and wires, and taken together, the many circuits the twelve major and multiple minor meridians make throughout the torso and limbs is called the Macrocosmic Orbit, or Large Circulation. (Figure 6.5)

So, to reiterate using the analogy of electrical wiring: The Conception Vessel—the enteric plexus—is the chi generator. The Governing Vessel—the central nervous sys-

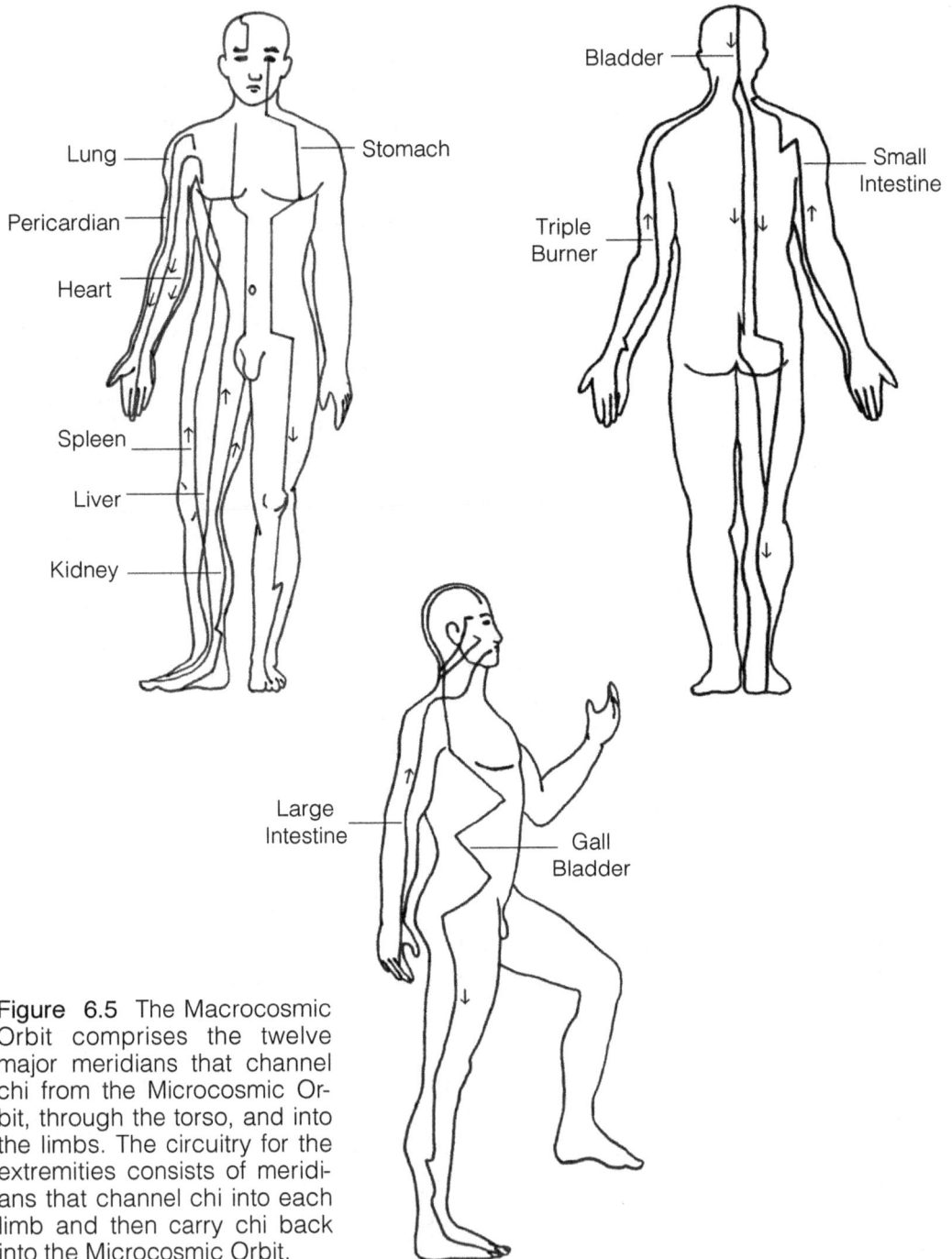

**Figure 6.5** The Macrocosmic Orbit comprises the twelve major meridians that channel chi from the Microcosmic Orbit, through the torso, and into the limbs. The circuitry for the extremities consists of meridians that channel chi into each limb and then carry chi back into the Microcosmic Orbit.

tem—is the chi switchboard/distribution center, the brain serving as the switchboard and the spine as the distributor. The circuit formed by the Conception and Governing Vessels is the Microcosmic Orbit, while the Macrocosmic Orbit is composed of the twelve major meridians that transmit the chi from the distributor (spine) into different neighborhoods—the torso and limbs. From there, the lines branch further into the numerous smaller wires that carry the chi into different homes—specific organs, tissue, and muscles—and finally to particular appliances—the cells.

The engine that powers the dynamo in the enteric plexus—the tantien—is the created by the natural processes of the peristaltic reflex caused by digestion, but again, the output of this process can be significantly amplified by rhythmic mechanical pressure applied downward upon the intestines by abdominal breathing. From the tantien, the chi is pushed into and through the central nervous system, where the switchboard (brain) causes some of it to be distributed (via the spine) to the various parts of the body along the wires of the peripheral nervous system and their surrounding meridians. The remainder of the chi not used elsewhere in the body travels through the brain then downward through the upper section of the Conception Vessel (the esophagus and stomach) and back into the tantien, where it joins with and is re-amplified by freshly generated chi to be recycled once again through the Microcosmic and Macrocosmic Orbits.

It is useful here to look at an interesting electromechanical device called a Van de Graaff generator. (Figure 6.6)

> A Van de Graaff generator is an electrostatic generator which uses a moving belt to accumulate very high amounts of electrical potential on a hollow metal globe on the top of the stand. It was invented by American physicist Robert J. Van de Graaff in 1929. The potential difference achieved in modern Van de Graaff generators can reach 5 megavolts. A tabletop version can produce on the order of 100,000 volts and can store enough energy to produce a visible spark.[38]

As you can see from the illustration, the functioning of the Van de Graaff generator has remarkable parallels to the functioning of the Microcosmic Orbit. In the figure, the Conception Vessel is 5 (esophagus, stomach) and 6 (tantien), and the Governing Vessel is 4 (spine) and 3 (brain). The yin/yang character of the resulting energy is obvious.

Because the brain is the main switchboard for sending bioelectrical impulses to be

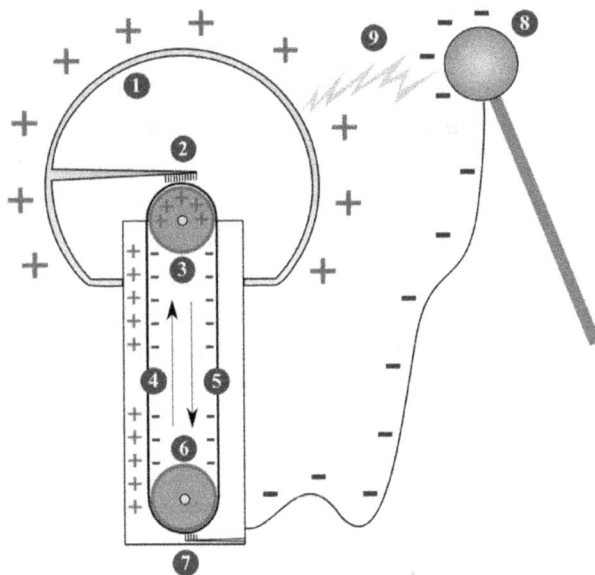

Figure 6.6 The operation of a Van de Graaff generator has remarkable parallels to the operation of the Microcosmic Orbit.[37]
1. Hollow metallic sphere (with positive charges)
2. Electrode connected to the sphere via a brush
3. Upper roller (nonmetallic)
4. Side of belt with positive charges
5. Side of belt with negative charges
6. Lower roller (metal)
7. Lower electrode (ground)
8. Spherical device with negative charges, used to discharge the main sphere
9. Spark produced by the difference of potentials

distributed, it is the principal destination for the bioelectricity flowing up the spine. Some of the bioelectrical distribution for the body—especially for the torso—is transmitted directly from the brain, but the bioelectrical flow up the spine also can be distributed, using mind intent, directly into the limbs at two major nerve branchings.

The branching into the legs occurs in the sacral region of the spine, just below the lumbar vertebrae. In Western medicine it is called the *sacral nerve plexus*, while in traditional Chinese medicine, the central acupuncture point in this area is called the *mingmen* point. The branching into the arms occurs at what Western medicine calls the *brachial nerve plexus*, which is represented in traditional Chinese medicine by the *dazhui* acupuncture point. The brachial plexus is located between the upper shoulder blades and extends down through each shoulder and into the arms. (Figure 6.7)

These two plexuses are critical to the Tai Chi chuanist. Dr. Becker has shown that, in terms of bioelectrical nerve circuitry, both plexuses have a positive electrical polarity, while the feet and hands have negative polarity.[39] Positive charges tend to migrate readily to areas of negative charge, and these two plexuses are the spots where the positively charged bioelectricity/chi flowing through the spine is impelled toward the ends of the limbs. This process occurs naturally, but it can be manipulated to send more energy than usual to the limbs.

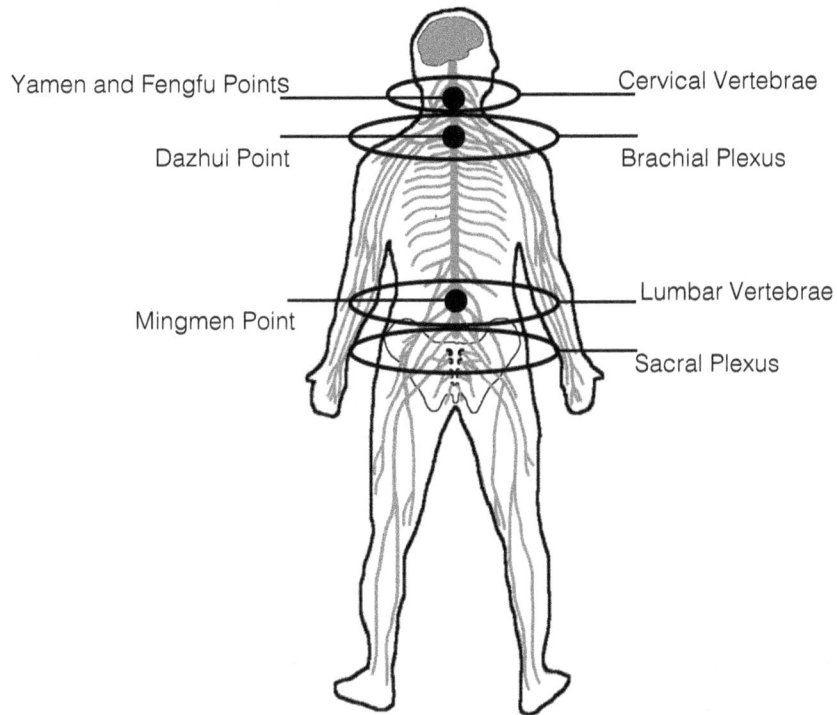

Yamen and Fengfu Points — Cervical Vertebrae

Dazhui Point — Brachial Plexus

Mingmen Point — Lumbar Vertebrae

Sacral Plexus

Figure 6.7 Important nerve plexus centers, spinal sections, and acupuncture points located along the Governing Vessel.

The manipulation begins when the Tai Chi exponent, using breathing and mind intent, diverts an extra-large pulse of bioelectrical/chi energy down the leg, all the way to the sole of the foot. Because of a combination of sinking onto the pushing leg, waist twisting, and the physiological configurations of both the outbound meridians and the fascial trains in the legs, this energy tends to spiral down around the leg, in one direction or another, to the sole. From there, through a combination of pushing upward through a gravity assist, waist twisting, and the physiological configurations of the inbound meridians and the fascial trains, the energy then spirals upward around the leg, in the opposite direction from which it spiraled down. It then surges into the pelvis and waist, where it is directed into the upper body. This downward and upward bouncing, spiraling surge has the physiological effect of increasing the muscular push from the leg and adding to the power generated by the superficial back and other fascial lines, and it also amplifies the energetic output by adding the bioelectric/bioelectromagnetic pulses locally created by the leg's muscular output.

Once this amplified rebounding energy surges upward into the spine, it can be manipulated at both the sacral and brachial plexuses. This is analogous to using a diverter valve to direct water flowing through a pipe into one or another pipe, and the manipulation depends on that important body alignment: a straightened spine or, more accurately, a straightened Governing Vessel. The practitioner is encouraged to tuck in his buttocks to cause his sacrum and tailbone to point downward instead of slightly back, which straightens the lumbar vertebrae. He also is encouraged to tuck in his chin slightly and pop out the inion, which straightens the neck. In the previous chapter, I discussed the impact that straightening these two vertebral sections has on the functioning of the Tai Chi bow, but to reiterate here:

When the Tai Chi player executes a particular force using the Tai Chi movements of Push or of Ward Off or Press in conjunction with Roll Back, the combined elements create a pulse or surge of elastic physical force and cause it to move upward from the leg, through the waist and torso, and into a particular upper body part. Straightening the curves of the lumbar and cervical vertebrae make it possible for that force to be directed properly and fully to the crown of the head, instead of exiting through the belly or neck.

That previous discussion regarded only the physical force of the movements, but the same paradigm holds true for chi energy, and ideally, both physical force and chi energy work in tandem. In other words, we want to pulse the chi energy into and rebound it out of only one leg at a time, then direct it through the waist and torso and into and through one arm, all in perfect coordination with bodily movements that do the same thing with physical force. Straightening the lumbar and cervical curves opens up the spine so that the chi rebounding up the spine can flow more readily through the Governing Vessel, but it also has the effect of giving one greater control over how much of the rebounding surge continues to flow through the Microcosmic Orbit and how much of it is directed into the limbs.

First we'll look at how the lumbar and sacral vertebrae—the waist, the commander—controls the rebounding flow of chi into the lower limbs and directs it more strongly into one or the other leg. This is a relatively straightforward process of tensing the muscles on one or the other side of these vertebral regions, and straightening and relaxing them on the other side. The tensing effect occurs naturally on the side of the supporting leg (yin side) due to the muscular contractions caused by the effort of carrying most of the body weight when in this posture, and

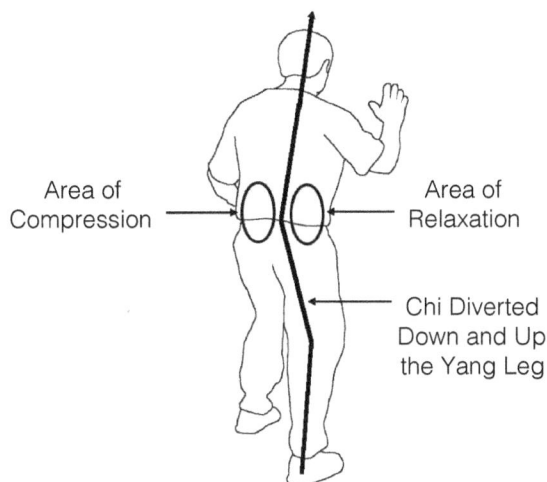

Area of Compression

Area of Relaxation

Chi Diverted Down and Up the Yang Leg

Figure 6.8 Brush Knee Twist Step showing chi flow to the legs. The body weight and posture naturally compress the muscles around the lumbar and sacral regions, sending more chi flow down and up the leg of the unweighted side.

this can be augmented by also intentionally tensing or compressing the muscles there.

The compressed muscles on that side impede the chi flow to the weight-bearing leg, causing the flow to course more readily down and up the opposite, pushing leg (yang side), whose channel is opened because of the slight stretching of the muscles on that side. (Figure 6.8) This combination diverts the extra-strength pulse going down the Governing Vessel/spine and into the yang leg and keeps the channel open as the energy rebounds upward, through waist and torso. It also is further evidence in the case against double-weighting because double-weighting precludes the proper energy flow by damming-off both sides at the same time, almost completely stagnating the chi flow and isolating the upper and lower body from each other.

Straightening the neck is critical to send the pulses of chi energy coming up the Governing Vessel/spine correctly into the arms. Under normal and relaxed circumstances, when the chi pulsing up the spine arrives at the brachial plexus, most of it continues to flow up through the neck, and into the brain. Some of it then continues over the top of the head and then downward into and through the Conception Vessel and on through another cycle in the Microcosmic Orbit. When the arms are at rest, a much smaller portion of the chi enters them at the brachial plexus. However, when you tuck in the chin and pop out the inion, you are able to tense the muscles around a closely-related pair of acupuncture points at the base of the neck called the *yamen* and *fengfu* points. These are the first and second acupuncture points, respectively, above the *dazhui* point, which is, again, the center of the brachial plexus.

No Compression

Undiverted Flow

Full-strength Flow

Lessened Flow

Area of Relaxation

Area of Compression

Diverted Flow

Full-strength Flow

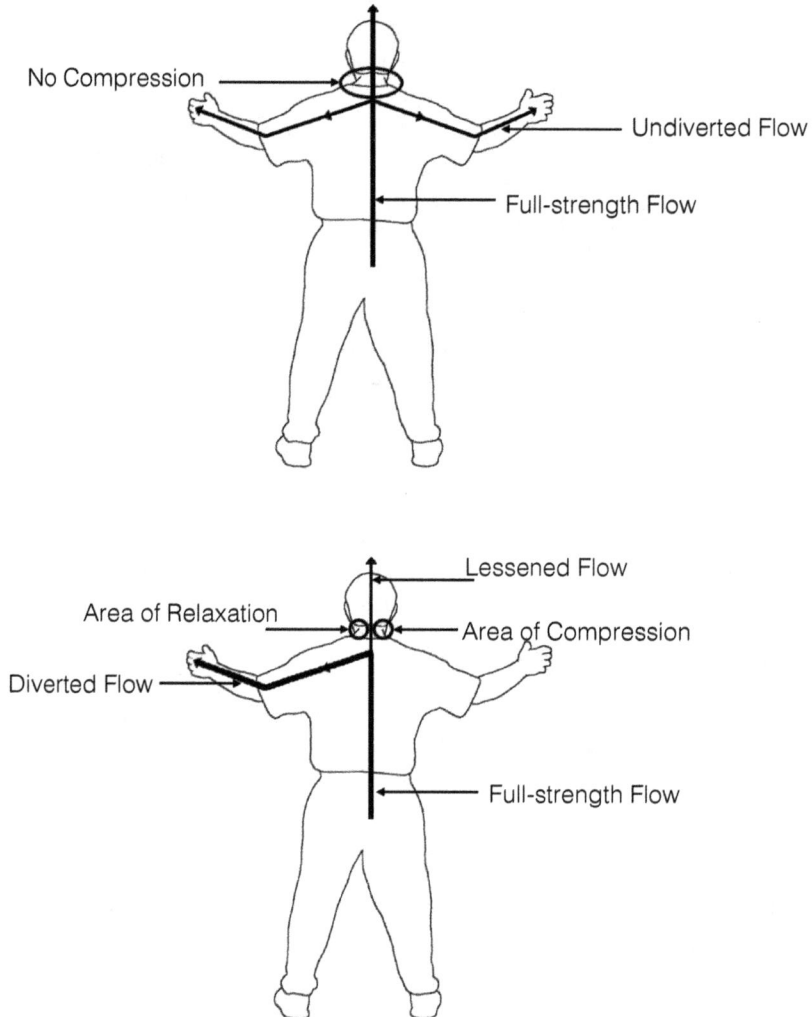

**Figure 6.9** When the muscles on both sides of the neck are relaxed, chi flows upward and equally through the arms. When the muscles on one side of the neck are compressed, more chi is diverted into the arm on the opposite side.

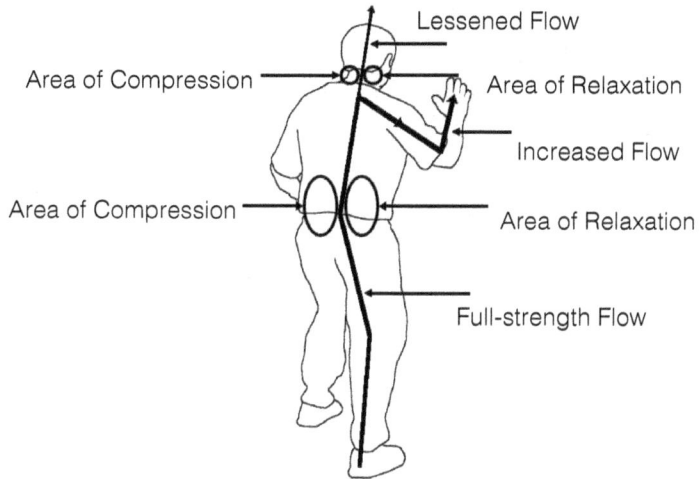

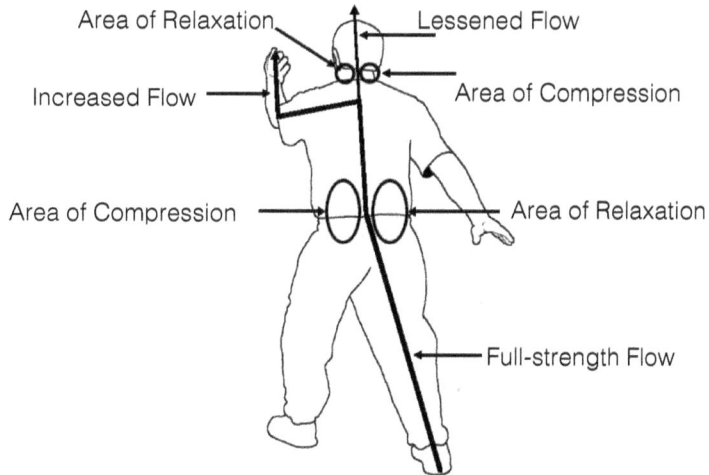

**Figure 6.10** Many Tai Chi movements entail compressing the muscles around the lumbar/ sacral region and the muscles around the cervical vertebrae to channel chi through specific limbs.

This tensing isn't rigid, but feels more like a moderate compression than like a clenching of the muscles. Tensing these muscles deliberately crimps the flow of chi there, causing the energy flowing upward to back up in the brachial plexus. Since it has nowhere else to go, the excess flow, which is highly positively charged, is diverted into the arms and impelled toward the negatively charged hands. The tensing is a very natural process that you can easily feel. Stand in the Open Tai Chi stance, but instead of lifting both hands, lift only one while paying attention to the muscles in question. You'll see that if you lift your right hand, the muscles on the left side of the neck will naturally compress slightly, and if you lift your left hand, the muscles on the right side will compress.

> Any [DC] electrical current grows weaker with distance, due to resistance along the transmission cable. The smaller the amperage and voltage, the faster the current dies out. Electrical engineers solve this problem by building booster amplifiers every so often along a power line to get the signal back up to strength. For currents measured in nano-amperes and microvolts, the amplifiers would have to be no more than a few inches apart —just like the acupuncture points! I envisioned hundreds of little DC generators like dark stars sending their electricity along the meridians, an interior galaxy that the Chinese had somehow found and explored by trial and error over two thousand years ago.
>
> –Robert O. Becker[40]

Tensing the muscles on both sides of the neck points sends the chi energy equally down both arms, but usually this might be considered a case of energetic double-weighting, stagnating the chi in both the upper limbs and making the upper body top-heavy with energy rather than light and flexible. But you can, in fact, deliberately tense the muscles on one side to inhibit the flow to that side and simultaneously stretch or open them on the other side to send more of the chi down that arm. (Figure 6.9) Tensing the muscles on the weighted side sends the energy down the arm on the unweighted side for Press movements, and tensing on the unweighted side sends the energy down the arm on the weighted side for Ward Off movements. (Figure 6.10)

We also can note that the opening and closing of these two sets of muscles help control the functioning of the Tai Chi bow by assisting in creating the elastic tension and relaxation required to draw and release the bow through activity of the fascial arm lines. The tensioning activity of the bow temporarily crimps the chi flow, so that when the crimp is released, the chi then pulses forward in a surge, along with the fascial snapping, into the receptor limb.

The energy flow works in two different ways with Push since Push is technically rolling the Tai Chi sphere straight forward and backward and cannot directly involve the twisting of Roll Back. There are two stances one can employ when using Push. The first is the common one, where one is in a bow stance and the energy is channeled through the leg and torso much as it is in Brush Knee Twist Step even though you're rolling the ball straight forward. The second is found primarily, it would seem, in Wu Family and Northern Wu styles, where the feet are evenly planted. The Push energy is sent down both legs at once, bounces back upward through the waist and spine, then shoots out of both arms simultaneously. (Alternatively, the energy coming up the spine can be coalesced around the brachial plexus for a Shoulder Strike using the upper back.)

Because this version of Push has an evenly weighted stance and uses equal energy flows in both arms at the same time, it would seem to be double-weighted in two different ways at once. However, this Push works and still utilizes the Tai Chi bow, and while it cannot express the long force because its stance isn't deep enough, it can express the short force with very jolting results. How can this be possible? Or rather, is it possible that a condition of double-double-weightedness can actually be a condition of single-weightedness, where all the elements of the bow are combined in one compound body movement?

Perhaps so. In this case, the two legs are both the stabilizer and one limb of the bow, the torso is the other limb of the bow, the two arms are twin arrows, and the tensioner is the sudden lowering of the weight followed by a simultaneous and rapid rebound (gravity assist) up both legs. The sudden free fall created by lowering the body weight provides the opportunity to open up the muscles on both sides of the sacral plexus, and by the time they are tightened again during the rebound to take up the body weight, the upward moving energy has already passed into the spine. From there, it shoots upward to the brachial plexus, only to be diverted strongly into both arms by a tensing of the muscles on both sides of the neck. Because the cervical vertebrae remain straightened, the fact that the chi is mostly diverted equally into both arms does not preclude the tensioning and release of both sides of the bow of the superficial back fascial line. And to validate this idea that double-double-weightedness can, at least sometimes, act as single-weightedness, think of a yin movement, such as the downward Pull after the initial lifting of the hands in Open

Tai Chi. In this movement, the legs are double-weighted and so are the arms, yet the Pull works for the same reason the Push does.

In the average person, the bioelectrical/bioelectromagnetic flow is of average strength and is, for the most part, entirely unconscious, but this doesn't have to be the case. Chi-building exercises, which include chi kung, yoga, and meditation as well as the several internal martial arts, give the practitioner tools to help improve posture and to deliberately release the tensions that inhibit the free flow of chi and, at the same time, amp-up the flow—often for self-defense, but always for health and personal development. As a chi-building exercise, Tai Chi has the fourfold function of increasing the generation of chi, making the exerciser more sensitive to it, teaching the exerciser to channel it in the body, not just more powerfully but with intent, and training the exerciser to deliberately manipulate it so that it can manifest in various ways.

Going back to the hydraulic analogy mentioned earlier, you can take a pipe of a given size (amperage) and open up the pressure all the way (raise the voltage); you can use a diverter valve to send the water more strongly through one or another side pipe; and you can attach different types of fixtures—faucet, spigot, shower head, dishwasher—to deliberately regulate and utilize the flow in various ways. But as with all analogies, the hydraulic analogy is not a completely accurate description. While the size of a pipe physically limits the amount of water flow, the flow of chi, being bioelectromagnetism, has no such limits. Thus, chi-building exercises can dramatically increase not just the chi's voltage, but its amperage as well, with no practical limit except for the exerciser's own limitations.

Sensitivity is simply learning to feel that flow within your own body through a process of improving body alignments, relaxing muscles and joints, and paying attention to the sensations within your own body. But it also might be that the higher amperages and voltages created by practicing Tai Chi open one's nervous system to a higher range of sensitivity to both internal and external stimulus than it might otherwise be aware of.

Tai Chi is often referred to as an "internal" martial art. The primary reason for this is that the practitioner emphasizes what is going on inside the body (chi flow, alignments, relaxation, etc.) over what what occurs on the outside of the body (muscular movement). Related to this is something alluded to in the Tai Chi Classics: Chi "adheres to the spine and back". Chi flowing up the spine lights up the spine with energy, and at the same time, it creates sort of a shell of chi surrounding the adept's dorsal, exterior side. The adepts ventral and vulnerable yin side—the interior side—is thus protected. Maybe it is not simply a comment on odd posture when Tai Chi's legendary founder, Chang-San-feng, is described as having a back rounded like a turtle's.

This turtle-back sensation is created energetically, not by tensing or arching the muscles of the back. Tensing or arching the back will, in fact, inhibit the chi flow. For the energy to flow up the back and accumulate there, the muscles of the back must be relaxed, opened, and expanded. In Tai Chi, the downward contraction of the abdominal muscles is what generates and impels the chi. Tai Chi—and all internal martial arts—emphasize the ventral musculature—the torso's yin side—to create power, while the external martial arts emphasize the dorsal musculature—the torso's yang side—the tensing of which automatically tenses the abdominal muscles, but in a different way than does the abdominal breathing of the internal martial arts.

# Energy Fields

**Now, let's look** at this energy system in another way. As noted earlier, the presence of electrical potential produces an electrical field, and any flow of electrical current produces an electromagnetic field that flows with the current. The fields that surround electrical power plants are spherical in shape (absent gravity and the presence of other electrical/electromagnetic/magnetic fields) and can have an effective diameter of a mile. Generally speaking (again, ignoring the effects of gravity and other fields), the electromagnetic field that surrounds a wire is tubular in shape as it follows the length of the wire, and it is much smaller in diameter than is a field that surrounds an electrical dynamo.

On a practical level, however, nothing in the universe—at least nothing that we know of—exists in such isolation that it isn't affected by gravity or by magnetic/electromagnetic fields produced, on the smaller scale, by living bodies or, on the larger scale, by astronomical bodies, from planets up to galaxies and galactic clusters. Magnetic and electromagnetic fields might be strongest around their sources, but theoretically, electromagnetic fields extend infinitely into space all around—even permeating most forms of solid matter. Of course, the effects of a given field are stronger close to the source and dissipate to inconsequential influence at greater ranges.

The electric/electromagnetic generating/distribution system of the human body is no different, and the body produces a number of fields that act and interact on several levels. On the larger scale, there is the whole-body field around the Microcosmic Orbit, which has both an active and a passive component, and on the smaller scale, there are the fields related to the Macrocosmic Orbit—the fields surrounding the meridians in the arms and legs.

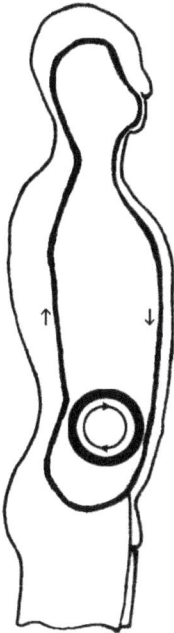

Figure 6.13 The rotating ball of energy in the belly powers the chi through the Microcosmic Orbit.

We'll start with the passive component of the field generated by the Microcosmic Orbit, which surrounds the generator of chi in the tantien: the enteric plexus. As discussed previously, over time, one develops the sensation of a mass of energy sunken and condensed within the gut, which I've termed the chi belly. (Figure 6.13) At first, this mass just seems static, but with attention and practice you learn that, by using reverse breathing, you can create a ball of energy in the middle of this mass. Once you can feel that ball, you can make it spin independently of the general condensed bioelectromagnetic energy in the tantien. Even without the sensation of this ball of energy, the body still produces most of its bioelectrical charge in the gut, but awareness of this ball can allow one to consciously increase the output because the breathing process that creates and rolls it further stimulates the production and mobilization of chi. This is why reverse breathing produces such powerful results.

The ball can be sent spinning forward or backward along any of the tangents defined by Push and Ward Off or around one side or the other by Press, but the forward orientation of the rotation is the norm because that synchronizes more naturally with the natural direction of the flow of chi through the Microcosmic Orbit and helps to properly propel the chi into the Governing Vessel. Rolling the energy ball backward reverses the chi flow, pulling it backward through the Microcosmic Orbit. This is necessary to do in brief instances for martial purposes, but as for making it as a regular, long-term practice, the reader might refer to the cautions about reverse breathing noted in the chapter on breathing, which I think also apply to frequently reversing the natural chi flow through the Microcosmic Orbit.

The chi ball in the gut is the rotor of the body's dynamo. This is an energetic matter, but if we think back on the Van de Graaff generator described in the previous section, the chi ball is like the lower pulley that drives the mechanism. And like any dynamo, the tantien is surrounded by an electrical field—electrical rather than electromagnetic because the tantien produces electrical potential, but the electrical potential simply cycles and does not move, and of course, electricity must be moving to produce an electromagnetic field.

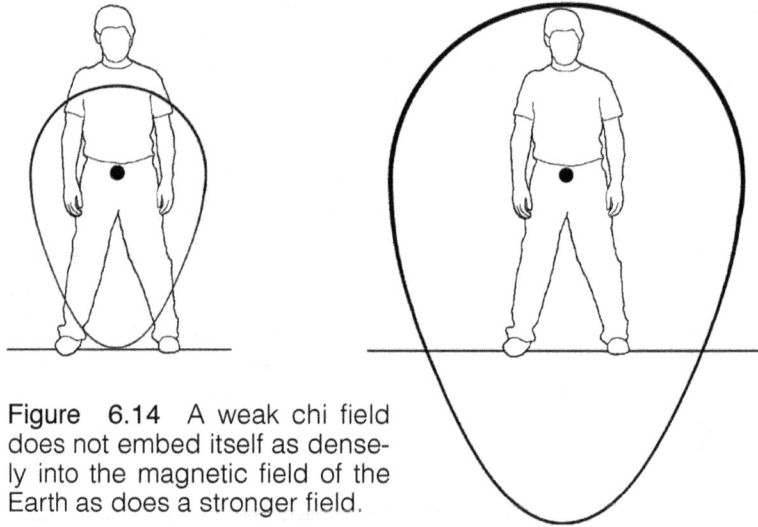

Figure 6.14 A weak chi field does not embed itself as densely into the magnetic field of the Earth as does a stronger field.

This might seem to be contradicted by the fact that the gut produces steady pulsations of bioelectricity along its length, which would instigate a bioelectromagnetic flow rather than a simple electric field. While this is technically the case, the convoluted configuration of the gut randomizes the direction of flow, much like the circuitry inside an electrical transformer or switching unit does. While there might be directional flows within segments of these convolutions, as a whole, the convolutions direct the flow this way and that instead of strictly linearly, and the compound effect is an electrical field instead of a steady linear electromagnetic flow.

This field is augmented by the electrical field that surrounds the brain. "As a side effect of the electrochemical processes used by neurons for signaling, brain tissue generates electric fields when it is active. When large numbers of neurons show synchronized activity, the electric fields that they generate can be large enough to detect outside of the skull, using electroencephalography or magnetoencephalography."[41] But this secondary field is much smaller than the one generated in the tantien because the brain does not produce bioelectricity in the same quantity that the enteric plexus does, functioning instead as a switchboard to simply direct it. Furthermore, the brain is just as convoluted as are the intestines, so as with the intestines, any linear flow of bioelectricity within it would be entwined enough to produce a field rather than a flow.

The fact that the compound field created by the enteric plexus and the brain is a bioelectric field and therefore does not move is the reason I refer to this aspect of the whole-body field as "passive." It is your whole-body field in a yin state of non-movement. Like the field around a dynamo, the passive field would be spherical in shape if it were not influenced by gravity or other fields. But gravity does pull on it, distending it downward into an egg-shape. This, I speculate, contributes to the ability of a Tai Chi exponent to root his energy—in this case, embedding his personal field deeply within both the Earth itself and the Earth's magnetic field. The more powerfully one can generate chi in the tantien, the denser the passive whole-body field will be. This means its effective range will be greater, enabling it to embed more deeply. It's the daruma doll idea on a larger, energetic scale. (Figure 6.14)

Now let's look at the active aspect of the whole-body field. The Microcosmic Orbit is not just the body's generating system—the enteric plexus—and the switchboard—the brain. It also contains two major transmission lines: one very powerful one up the spine, and one of lesser energy down through the esophagus and stomach. In these, the bioelectricity flows linearly, producing a complete circuit between the tantien and brain—and with that circuit, an electromagnetic field. This effectively turns the entire body into a large, if weak, bioelectromagnet, with the tantien being the negative pole and the brain being the positive pole. Because it is a bioelectromagnetic field, it has motion, and thus is the yang, active element of the whole-body field.

As with all such fields produced around a magnetic or electromagnetic object, the magnetic lines of force radiate out of the magnet's positive pole, circle in all directions around the magnet, and reenter it at the negative pole. We can see this in visual representations of such fields, be they around simple bar magnets or around more complex magnetic structures, such as the Earth. (Figure 6.15) When considering the magnetic field that surrounds the Earth, called the "magnetosphere" and which is produced by geodynamism rather than by electrical flow, it is useful to note that what we normally think of as the Earth's north pole is really its negative pole. That's why the positive end of a magnetized needle in a compass will point in that direction, since, with magnetism, opposites attract and likes repel. Maybe we ought, like the ancient Chinese, to orient maps with the South Pole at the top.

So the flow of bioelectricity through the Microcosmic Orbit produces an electromagnetic field whose lines of force radiate upward along the spine, then fountain out through the body's positive pole at the crown of the head (also referred to as the "crown chakra"). From there, it flows around the outside of the body and reenters the body's negative pole at the perineum (also called the "root of life chakra"). (Figure 6.16)

The spine itself is the axis of the field because that is where the bioelectricity

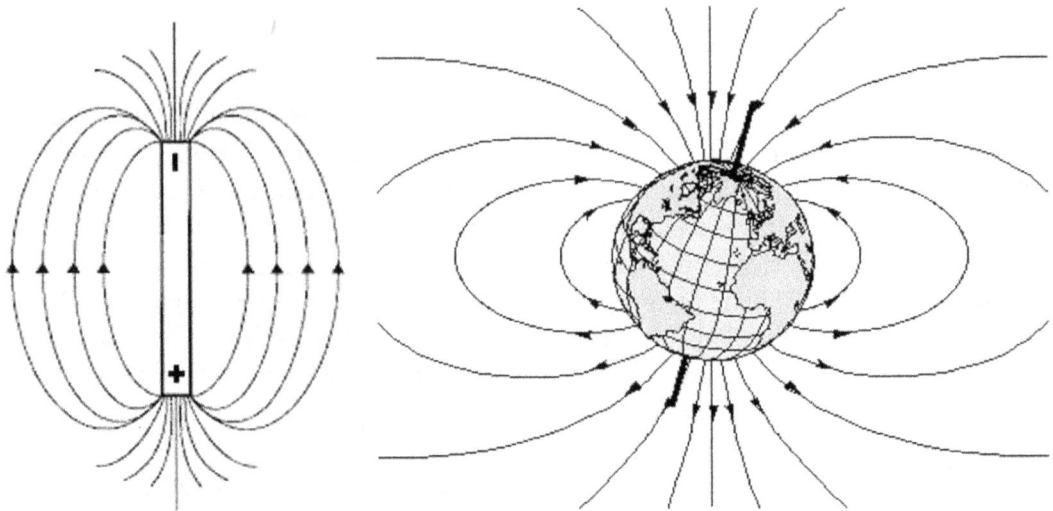

Figure 6.15 Magnetism in a bar magnet (left) is caused by an alignment of the iron molecules in a common direction. Magnetism in the Earth is produced by geodynamic processes.

that is generated in the gut subsequently flows the strongest as it is pushed through the densely massed neurons of the relatively narrow spinal column. In fact, the small entry point into the Governing Vessel from the Conception Vessel—the sacrum—acts much like a nozzle attached to a hose, condensing the relatively diffuse electromagnetic surge developed in the Conception Vessel into a much more powerful pressure in the spine. Again, this is the reason that amped-up chi flow seems to "light up" the spine and brain, and also why it is said that "chi adheres to the back." We can see, as well, why an upright posture is important—otherwise, your polarity doesn't run straight up and down but is bent, unbalancing your field in relation to the magnetic field and gravitation of the Earth and weakening its power in the process.

It is important to restate that the whole-body field or its parts—active and passive—do not actually have boundaries as shown in the illustrations. Instead they, like other fields, potentially extend infinitely and equally in all directions, although they are warped and influenced not just by gravity, but also all around by the fields of other living creatures, human-made electrical and electromagnetic sources, and large deposits of iron and water in or on the Earth. Such fields also are influenced by the fields of the Earth itself and of other astronomical bodies that produce magnetospheres—the Moon, Mercury, and Mars, for example, do not because their cores are

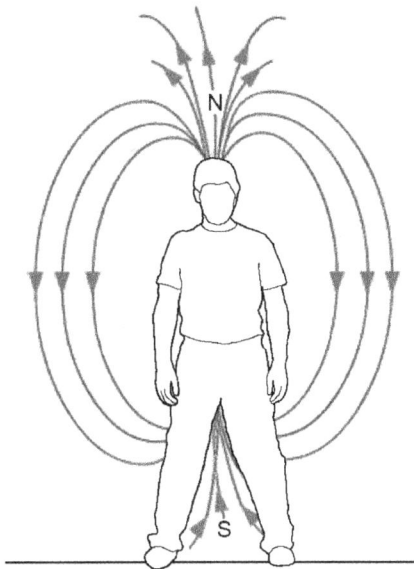

Figure 6.16 The electromagnetic chi field exhibits polarity and extends infinitely in all directions but is most powerful in proximity to the body.

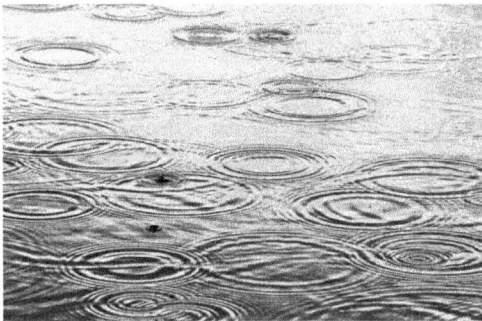

Figure 6.17 Raindrops on water create overlapping waves of energy in two dimensions. Imagine this effect spherically surrounding every source of magnetism and electromagnetism in three dimensions throughout the entire universe.

solidified rather than being rotating spheres of molten iron, and so there is no geodynamic effect. The sun also generates a huge electromagnetic field, as do other large astronomical structures, from gas giants (Jupiter, Saturn, etc.) to galaxies and black holes. Magnetic and electromagnetic fields are influenced by solar winds, as well, manifesting the visible waves of the auroras.

The entire universe, in fact, is awash in electromagnetic fields whose overlappings are mind-bogglingly complex. (Figure 6.17) However, an individual's field would be densest and less affected by other fields in the area immediately surrounding the body—less affected, at least, by smaller fields or weaker emanations from powerful but distant sources, all of which end up seeming like a random, generalized background field or flux. This background field or flux, as pervasive as the cosmic background microwave radiation that cosmologists believe is a remnant of the Big Bang, is the universal chi. One can consider one's own field, which is embedded within the universal chi, to be at its most powerful within the physical limits of arm's reach, for it is in this region that one can most directly influence it.

In *The Wellspring*, I discussed the idea that a more sensitive and powerful whole-body field would allow a Tai Chi adept to sense the fields of opponents and, to a greater or lesser degree, manipulate those fields for defense and attack. In other words, before bodies collide, energy fields merge. The Tai Chi Classics state that a "master senses an attack before it is launched— when the attack is just an idea in the mind of the attacker, but before he has acted on the idea." As the idea of an attack arises in the attacker's mind, it causes neurons to fire in his central nervous system, producing perturbations in his active biofield —perhaps in the specific area he intends to use, such as an arm and a fist—and the sensitive Tai Chi adept actually feels the change, whose impulses move at light speed and affect his own field before the attacker's body, moving far slower, has had a chance to act on the impulse.

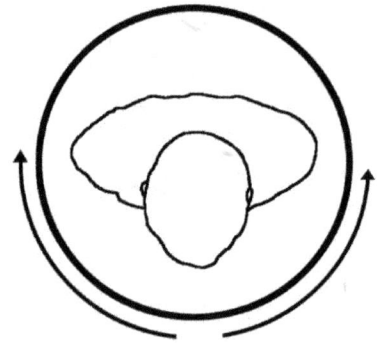

Figure 6.18 Roll Back spins incoming force around the defender's sides.

In Tai Chi, there is the concept of "hearing" one's opponent's energy with one's skin, and that is exactly what is happening here. This sensing occurs in the passive—yin—portion of the biofield since passivity gives rise to sensitivity and also because the passive field is related to the sensory apparatus of the autonomic nerves and the inbound meridians, whose first physical line of sensation is the skin. The Tai Chi adept would then be able to appropriately energize the active—yang—portion of his field, which is related to the action apparatus of the somatic nerves and the out-bound meridians. This allows the adept to respond to the attack, even as the attacker is launching his attack, with a fully charged active field augmented by superior balance and training in sophisticated body movements. Together, the sensing and subsequent action is a case of the quiescence of wu chi turning into the activity of tai chi. As the Tai Chi Classics say: "If my opponent does not move, I do not move. If my opponent moves, I move first."

And remember: If you can manipulate your own field, you can potentially affect the field of another—in essence, spinning or bouncing it off the mass of your denser chi field, causing part of your field to penetrate it either bluntly or sharply, or otherwise exploiting it. The simplest manipulation might be to avoid an attack by turning it to one side or the other, spinning the incoming force off the outside of the field by using Roll Back. (Figure 6.18) You also might bounce your field against that of your opponent. As with two inflated balls thrown toward each other, the one that has the most inflation and greater inner density will bounce the other ball away. Ward Off bounces the entire field diagonally across the body, Push

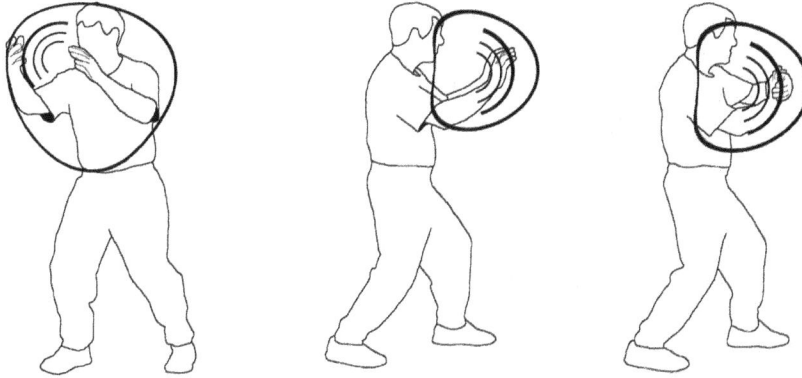

Figure 6.19 Ward Off (left) can produce an upward and outward surge diagonally through the chi field, Push (center) can produce a forward surge or bounce of energy straight forward in the center of the chi field, and Press (right) can produce a forward-bouncing compression of energy through one side of the chi field.

bounces the energy either forward or downward through center of the field, and Press bounces the energy through one side of the field. (Figure 6.19)

Obviously it would pretty magical to be able to use only one's energy fields against an attack, and maybe there are rare individuals out there whose expertise is so great that they can actually do that. But even for us folks of lesser skill, the fields and the physical movements can augment one another to dramatically increase our power. We'll look at that later, but first, we have to look at the interactions of different chi fields produced by the body. This becomes quite interesting because the complexity of human anatomy—particularly the articulation of the arms—means that energetically complex permutations are possible. Let's begin this part of the discussion by looking at how the chi force travels in the human body.

The easy answer is that it moves through the meridians of the Macrocosmic Orbit. In the legs, the meridians branching from the sacral plexus carry the flow down the outside of the legs to the soles, where it rebounds up the insides of the legs and back into the Microcosmic Orbit at the sacral plexus. In the arms, the flow is just the opposite. From the brachial plexus, it moves outward along the inside of the arms from shoulders to fingertips, then inward along the outsides of the arms and back through the shoulders into the Microcosmic Orbit at the brachial plexus. (It is helpful in this context to reexamine Figure 5.2 on pages 142–143 showing the fasciae of the arms, which run contiguously with the arm nerves and meridians and function in conjunction with them.)

Just as the bioelectrical flow through the main circuit of the Microcosmic Orbit creates the whole-body active field, the flow through the lesser circuits of the Macrocosmic Orbit also produces lesser fields, or sheathes of bioelectromagnetism, around each limb. The flow of the fields in the legs works in the same direction as the flow of the body's whole chi field: up through the inside of the legs then down through their outsides. (Figure 6.20) So, the flow in the legs works in conjunction with the whole body flow to lend stability and rooting and to produce power. However, the flow of the field around the arms runs in the opposite direction: outward through the inside of the arms then inward through their outsides.* (Figure 6.21) It is this oppositional flow in the arms, along with the arms' articulations, that can create a great number of energy dynamics within the whole-body chi field.

We'll look at how this might be in a moment, but first, it is interesting to note that the outbound flow of chi in the arms is associated not only with the in-

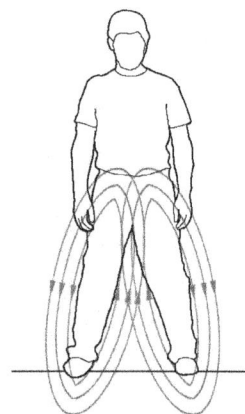

Figure 6.20 The chi in the legs flows in the same direction as the flow of the whole-body chi.

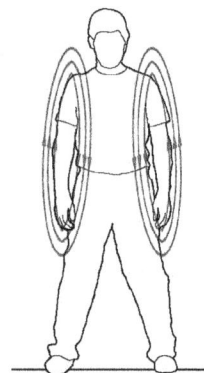

Figure 6.21 The chi in the arms flows in the opposite direction to the flow of the whole-body chi.

---

* It is interesting to note that the outbound flow of chi in the arms is associated not only with the insides of the arms, but also with the thumb, forefinger, and their half the middle finger, which are enervated by the same set of nerves, while the inbound flow of chi is associated with the outsides of the arms and with the ring and pinky fingers and their half of the middle finger, which are enervated by a separate set of nerves. This is why in Pull/Pluck, Pluck entails an active grasping with the thumb and first two fingers, while Pull entails a passive grasping with the last three fingers. (See the Pull/Pluck section in the chapter on the Ordinal Energies.)

Elementary physics told me that the currents and their associated electromagnetic fields would have to be affected in some way by external fields. In engineering terms, the biomagnetic fields would be coupled to the DC currents [produced by the body]. Hence charges impressed upon it by external fields would be "read out" rough perturbations in the current. Outside fields would also couple directly to the currents themselves, without acting though the biofields as intermediary, especially if the currents were semiconducting. In short, all living things having such a system would share the common experience of being plugged in to the electromagnetic fields pf earth. which in turn vary in response to the moon and sun.

—Robert O. Becker[43]

sides of the arms, but also with the thumb, forefinger, and half of the middle finger, which are enervated by the same set of nerves as the outbound flow. The inbound flow of chi is associated with the outsides of the arms and with half of the middle finger, the ring finger, and the pinky finger, which are energized by the same nerves as the inbound flow. This is why in Pull/Pluck, Pluck entails an active grasping with the thumb and first two fingers, while Pull entails passive grasping with the last three fingers. (See the Pull/Pluck section in the chapter on the Ordinal Energies.)

Regarding the energy dynamics of the chi flow in the arms in relation to the flow in the body, when the arms are hanging down at one's sides, the flow in them runs in opposition to the flow of the active whole-body field, whose energy fountains upward through the middle of the body then cascades downward around the outside of the body. So, when the arms are in their relaxed positions at one's sides, their inside surfaces carry a downward flow that is embedded in the active whole-body field's upward flow through the torso. Likewise, the arms' outside surfaces carry an upward flow that is embedded in the downward flow around the outside of the whole-body field. In magnetism, like polarities repel and opposite polarities attract, so this posture, with opposite polarities lying contiguously with each other, is not only relaxed in a muscular sense, it is energetically very stable and neutral.

This neutral condition changes, however, as soon as one lifts a hand. Lifting an arm, say, until it is parallel to the ground means that, energetically, one is now inserting a bar of horizontal flow through the middle of your whole-body field's verti-

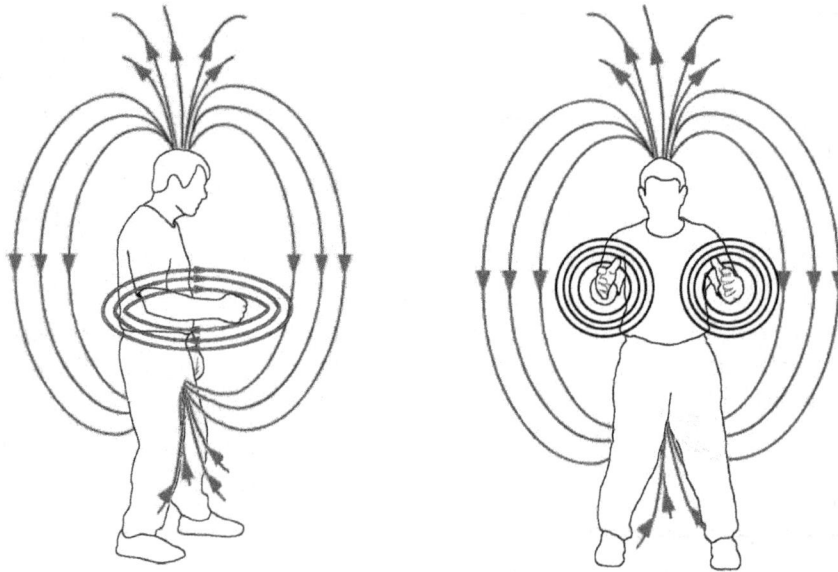

Figure 6.22 Lifting one arm parallel to the ground inserts a bar of chi flow perpendicular to the flow of the vertically oriented whole-body field. Lifting two arms introduces two separate and roughly parallel flows perpendicular to the vertical flow.

cal flow. (Figure 6.22) Lifting two arms introduces two separate and roughly parallel horizontal flows into the whole-body field's vertical flow. If you hold your arms still, the flows are just flows, but if you begin waving the arms around, their bioelectromagnetic influences will create currents within the whole-body chi field—both the active and passive parts. It is like standing neck-deep in water and waving your arms around, causing currents, swirls, and eddies. And just as you can feel the pressure of the water increase on one side of your arms and decrease on the other when you wave them in water, if you are relaxed enough, you can feel the pressure of the biofield increase and decrease on your arms when you wave them around in it. Again, this is "hearing" chi energy with your skin, but in this case, you are sensing your own energy field, not that of an opponent as described above.

Most arm movement is relatively random—reaching for a glass of water or smoothing down your hair—so the currents their movements create are random and transient. But the movements of Tai Chi, which emulate the dynamics of the tai chi symbol as explicated in the chapters on the Thirteen Postures, generate more-purposeful currents that can be used to create wavelike force, swirls, or vortex-like suction within the whole-body field. And the more powerful the biofield of the person who creates the waves and swirls, the more powerful those waves and swirls will be in their effects on other fields. These waves have to be caused by intentionally directed movements rather than random ones because random movements don't create powerful pulses of bioelectric energy in the limbs as do intentionally directed movements and so have less energetic impact on the field. Back to water: It's a little like the difference between creating a slight current by just reaching out as opposed to deliberately and forcefully waving a flexible skin-diving flipper in the water, which will produce and transmit a far bigger wave of energy. And just like a purposeful current created in water can be felt by someone standing close by, so too can purposeful currents in biofields be felt by others, whether they consciously sense them or not. This accounts for the sense of "presence" that surrounds expert adepts.

In fact, through correct movement, the interactions of the bioelectromagnetic fields around your arms can create an energetic subfield between your arms that becomes independent of the general whole-body field. To examine this, we need to look at how we can alter what happens to the energy flowing down the arms. When the hand is in its normally relaxed posture, the wrist is held straight, though not rigidly so, and the chi flows unimpeded down through the inside of the arm, through the palm, then into the fingers. When it reaches the fingertips, it flows back toward the shoulder through the outsides of the fingers, the back of the hand, and the outside of the arm. (Figure 6.23) This way of holding the wrist is called the Lady-like Wrist, and some Tai Chi stylists—notably Cheng Man-ching—advocate its use in the striking hand of Brush Knee Twist Step during form practice rather than the cocked-back wrist more commonly seen because the posture of Lady-like Wrist allows the chi to move unimpeded completely through the Nine-Channel Pearl, all the way to the tips of the fingers.

But cocking back the wrist has a functional aspect. When you do so, the cocked wrist creates a kink in the chi flow. Some of the chi still circulates normally through the hand and fingers, but the build-up caused by the kink causes some of the chi to flood into, coalesce in, and then exude from the heart of the palm. (Figure 6.24) This exuded chi is what can, using the short force, penetrate into the opponent in open-palm and other strikes. It often is noted that the heart of the palm of the striking hand of Brush Knee Twist Step feels like it "pops" out at the apex of the strike. This sensation is caused by the condensed, backed-up chi being jolted into and out of the palm.

Chi emanating, rather than jolting, from the two palms can create an interest-ing and easy-to-feel effect. Stand with your feet about hip-width apart, and move your hips and waist in the figure-eight pattern previously discussed in the section on Chan-ssu Chin. As you do, hold both forearms comfortably out in front of you and roll them with the waist and hip move-ment, describing a sphere in front of you that is held between the palms. (Figure 6.25, and also see Figure 2.26, page 50.) In the beginning, you can hold a real ball—one about the size of a soccer ball—to establish the rolling effect, but you can quick-ly dispense with the real ball in lieu of the tangible sensation of the chi ball that will develop.

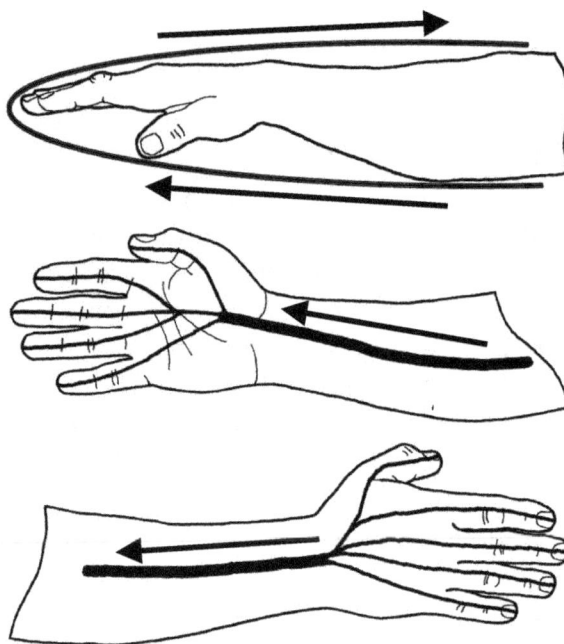

Figure 6.23 In the hand posture Ladylike Wrist, chi flows down through the inside of the arm, cycles around the tips of the fingers, then returns to the body through the outside of the arm.

After a time—usually rela-tively short—you will actually be able to feel the sensation of holding and rolling a sphere of energy between your hands. This sensation is caused by the interaction of the bioelectromagnetic energy that is coursing down the insides of the arms and exuding from both palms. Since this energy is positive in polarity in both palms, the resulting sensation is like the repulsing force you feel when you push together the positive poles of two magnets because that's exactly what's happening. The stronger your chi, the stronger the repulsing force feels and the more energetically "solid" the ball will be.

The diameter of this sphere can be as large as you can comfortably reach—from about the crown of the head to the tantien—or it can be small. Large hip/waist ro-tation produces a larger sphere, and the larger the sphere is, the more tenuous it will feel. Decreasing the size of the hip/waist rotation also decreases the size of the sphere between your hands. With very small hip/waist rotation, you can make this

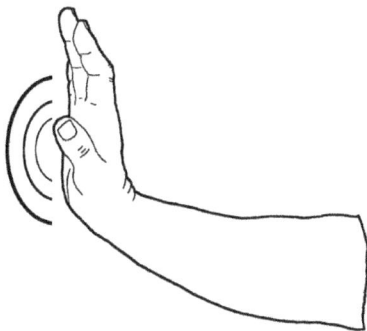

Figure 6.24 In an open-palm strike, the bent wrist causes a kink in the chi flow, accumulating some of the chi in the hand and exuding it from the palm.

sphere as small as a marble, as small as a pea. The smaller you make it, the more the wrists cock back, which forces more of the chi flow into your palms, making this smaller sphere feel warmer and more solid. Of course, this sphere is the same one mentioned at the beginning of this book.

Let's think of what is happening on an energetic level when you create this sphere. You are generating a rotating sphere of bioelectromagnetic energy held between your palms that, as it rotates, becomes divorced from your whole-body field. This spherical field is encased in your general field, but it commands an ever-shifting polarity in relation to the whole-body field, which maintains a fixed vertical polarity. It is as if a current in a stream has created an eddy that takes on an independent existence or vitality that is no longer driven by the main current but just rotates within it.

Simply rolling the ball side to side doesn't produce an energy wave, just an action potential. It is like an electrical generator that doesn't have anything plugged into it. But the many, varied, and coordinated swirling arm movements of the Eight

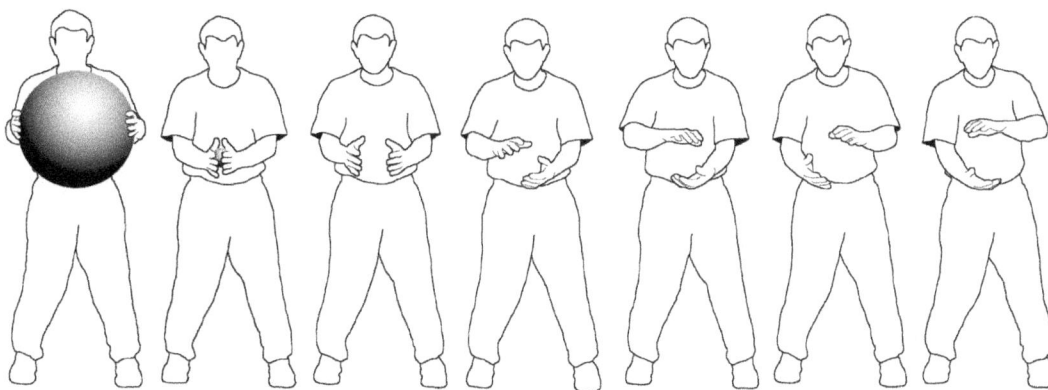

Figure 6.25 Chi exuding from the palms exerts a repelling sensation like that caused by pushing two magnets together at their positive (or negative) poles. Rolling the hands around in a circle causes this sensation to feel like rolling a ball between one's hands.

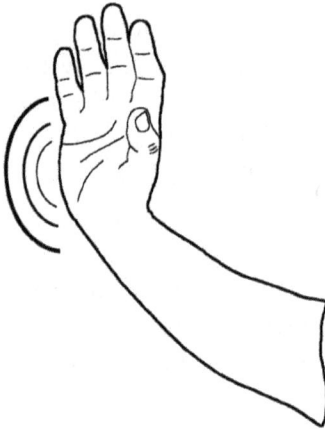

Figure 6.26 The roof-tile palm channels the chi flow into and through the edge of the heel of the hand.

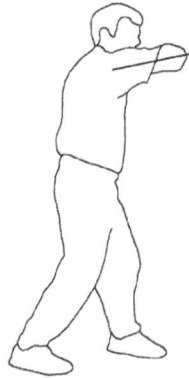

Figure 6.27 Cocking back the elbow crimps the chi flow and sends some of it out the end of the elbow.

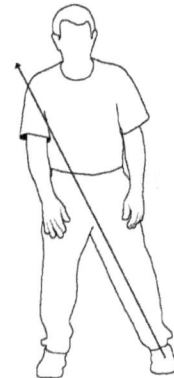

Figure 6.28 Chi can be channeled straight from the foot, into the shoulder.

Gates can transform the action potential into complex currents in the whole-body chi field that can be used to manipulate both one's own field and the field of an opponent. Relaxation is key. Making your arms rigid or muscularly tight can't do the trick because then the chi won't properly flow through them to form the vibrant bars of energy required to manipulate the whole-body field into whirls and eddies. Muscular tension won't work also because it makes the arm more densely solid, and dense solids can't cause whirls or eddies as readily as can more diffuse objects. One way to look at this is that, electrically, people with less resistance (fewer Ohms, in electrical terms) are the better conductors.

Remember: You can create a far bigger wave of energy in water by waving a flexible, light-weight flipper than you can by waving a heavier but rigid iron bar. Using flexibility and softness allows you to create swirls and eddies and also pulses of energy that move through a larger field like a wave. This wave can be gentle and pushing or jolting and penetrating—again, the result is not from how much you tense the muscles or how hard you push, but from how round or flat you make the circles/ovals of the Cardinal Energies and how sharply you draw the energy back around their curves and recurves. The slower and more rounded the drawing back, the blunter the energy; the quicker and more acute the drawing back, the sharper the energy.

The energy flowing down the arm can be blocked at various spots to deliberately accumulate chi. Above are described Ladylike Wrist and the posture of the wrist during a standard palm strike. The wrist also can be twisted slightly as it cocks back, presenting the heel of the palm, called the Roof Tile Palm. (Figure 6.26) In this configuration, the energy coming down the arm exudes from a smaller area on the side of the heel of the palm for a sharp and targeted strike. The energy can be blocked at the elbow by cocking back the elbow for an elbow strike (Figure 6.27), or at the shoulder if you simply channel it to the shoulder and stop it there. (Figure 6.28) Or the energy can be led around in various circles and arcs, to redirect it, cycle it for throws, or tie it up, via the limits of human physiology, into joint locks. These ideas will be discussed below in greater detail.

One final note before we move on. Some Tai Chi masters recommend that you begin your form by facing north. This might be because that would align the positive pole of the natural cyclical flow of your personal active field with the negative pole of the Earth's magnetosphere, making for an energetically stable relationship between the fields of the practitioner and the Earth. However, this would only align the two fields at Open Tai Chi and Close Tai Chi since the body makes many turns and faces many directions during the performance of the set. But perhaps this alignment would be more important when doing chi kung exercises, which don't tend to deviate or turn much from the direction in which they begin. I've found, for example, that when I'm doing free-form Chan-ssu Chin, no matter which direction I start facing, my body will naturally gravitate to face north.

It is through your hands that you express your will, whether for martial arts, for health, or for healing. Your hands are the farthest point to which your Chi moves inside your body, and how they are held, and whether any muscles are tensed, influences the flow of energy.

—Yang Jwing-ming[42]

# Energy Manipulations

**In the previous** sections of this chapter, we looked at how chi is created and directed inside the body, how energy fields are created, and how the movement of the arms can manifest currents within the whole-body field. In this section, we'll examine how chi energy can be manipulated and utilized.

In the chapter on the Thirteen Postures, we saw how the pure circles of the Cardinal Energies define the four basic planes of movement the human body is capable of producing. We then saw how flattening the circles into ovals produces more powerful results. In that chapter, I restricted the actions of the spheres/ovals, basically, to the physicality of whole-body movements as expressed through the arms, but we can extrapolate this further to take in the whole-body energy system thanks to the idea that the chi flow in the arms can create currents, waves, swirls, and vortices in the whole-body field. To start this discussion, let's look at the physical phenomenon of waves to see how two separate energies working sympathetically or antagonistically can produce different effects.

Greatly simplified, a waveform is the transport of regularized disturbances or oscillations through a medium or through space. Mechanical waves, such as ocean waves, shock waves, and sound waves propagate through and distort a medium. There also are gravitational waves, which move through and distort gravitational fields, and gravity can distort tangible matter as evidenced by the tidal bulge produced by the Moon on the Earth's geophysical structure as well as on its surface water. Interestingly, waves that pass through a medium do not move the medium itself, but they do affect the medium energetically, as anybody who has ever listened to music, felt a shock wave, or stood in ocean waves before they break at a beach can testify. And while we usually think of mechanically produced waves moving through a medium, there are waves referred to as standing waves that do not move through their medium but remain stationary, either because the medium through which the wave travels is moving at the same speed but in the opposite direction or because the medium terminates on both ends, like a vibrating guitar string.

Electromagnetic waves are different from mechanically produced waves in that they travel through most physical matter as well as through a vacuum, but they do not directly act energetically upon physical objects through which they pass. They do, however, affect magnetic and electromagnetic fields and other electromagnetic waves that they encounter. Further, waves "can be transverse or longitudinal, depending on the direction of the oscillation. Longitudinal waves occur when the oscillations are parallel to the direction of propagation (the direction of energy transfer). An example is waves traveling through water. Transverse waves occur when a disturbance creates oscillations that are perpendicular to the propagation. An example is the tubular electromagnetic field surrounding an electrical line. While mechanical waves can be both longitudinal and transverse, all electromagnetic waves are transverse in free space."[44]

The actions and interactions of waveforms can be incredibly complex, as we noted in the previous section, and there are many types of waveforms, but my purpose here is not to explicate their entire range (which is way out of my league, anyway), but to use the most basic waveform—the sine wave—to illustrate a point. A sine wave is a regular undulation whose wavelength and amplitude remain constant. (Figure 6.29) In other words, the distance from one peak to the next is always the same, and, if the sine wave is centered on a horizontal line, all the crests of the wave are of equal height, and that height is exactly equal to the distance from the horizontal line to the bottoms of all the troughs of the wave. Interestingly, the recurved line through the middle of the tai chi symbol is a sine wave.

A single sine wave with a given wavelength and amplitude can be greatly affected by a second, overlapping sine wave of equal wavelength and amplitude. If the peaks and troughs of the two waves align perfectly, the effective energy of the two waves is doubled. If they are only partially in sync, the amplitude is greater than, but not double, that of one of the waves alone. And if they are perfectly misaligned, with the peaks of the first wave occurring at the troughs of the second wave, the energy of the two waves is effectively cancelled out. (A case of energetic double-weighting!) (Figure 6.30)

Now, let's return to the Cardinal Energies to examine how they work in con-

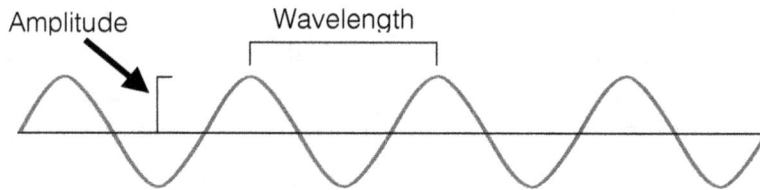

**Figure 6.29** A basic standing sine wave showing wavelength and amplitude.

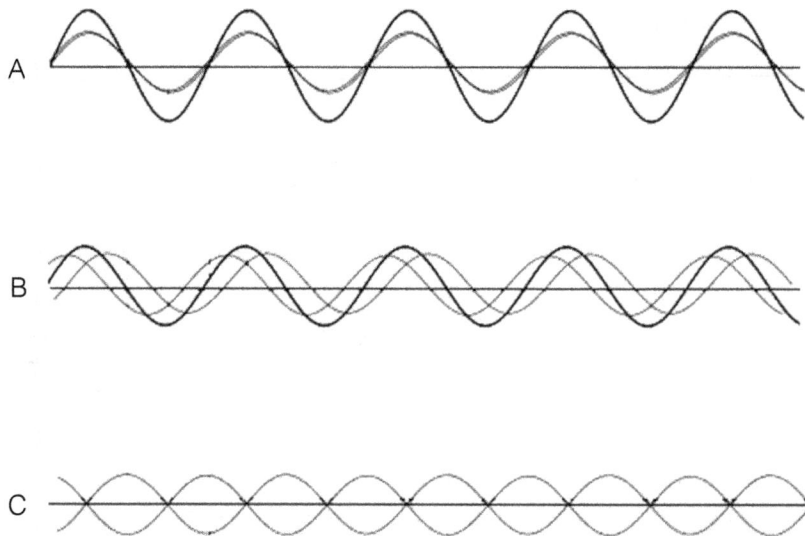

**Figure 6.30** Two identical sine waves traveling in opposite directions can have different interactions depending on their synchronization. A: Two waves perfectly synchronized produce a gestalt amplitude that is higher than either sine wave alone. B: Two waves in partial sync produce a somewhat lesser amplification. C: Two sine waves in complete opposition cancel each other.

junction with the whole-body field. As stated previously, an important precept in Tai Chi is that one should move the body as a single unit. This whole-body movement is not rigid, but is flexible, as is evident in the twisting and torquing provided by Roll Back and in the functioning of the Tai Chi bow, which utilizes the major fasciae to create an elastic connection between the lower and upper body. These give the body its physical force (as opposed to muscular strength), and can, in self-defense situations, produce Tai Chi's whipping/jerking/repelling power. But the whole-body aspect of the Tai Chi movements isn't limited to just the physicality of the body's movements. Because all parts of the body produce bioelectromagnetic fields, the movements of the body cause the fields of those parts that are in motion to operate with or upon the whole-body field.

Notice in the illustrations in the previous section how the whole-body field fountains up the spine than cascades down around the body. This is the field's natural cyclical flow, and it is oriented vertically. Thus, the Tai Chi adept can employ two of the three vertically oriented Cardinal Energies—Push and Ward Off—to directly exploit this cyclical flow. Exploiting the cyclical flow is limited to these two Cardinal planes because they, like the whole-body field, have a vertical orientation centered on the body's core—Central Equilibrium. Press and Roll Back operate differently, and we'll look at them shortly.

In exploiting the cyclical flow, the adept doesn't usually alter the directional flow of the field, except for brief moments. Instead, the adept uses mind intent, which we discussed in a different context elsewhere. The Tai Chi Classics make it clear that the attention the practitioner pays to what is going on inside the body—or on the whole-body field, which is certainly a more esoteric level than the simply physical—is as important, if not more so, than exactly how the body executes its physical movements. After all, a given Tai Chi movement might be performed somewhat differently in the various Tai Chi styles yet still be martially effective. Initially, this attention to the inner aspects focuses on the physical: body alignments, sinking the body weight into the legs, loosening the upper body, and so forth. After a time, as these elements become more ingrained in one's movement patterns, other aspects become apparent that couldn't be observed before. It's a lot like traveling across the country and approaching a mountain range—you can't see the territory that lies beyond until you climb and cross the mountains.

The first territory you come to after crossing the mountains of the purely physical aspects of Tai Chi consists of sensing the flow of chi throughout the body. First one begins to feel little surges or tinglings in different body parts here and there during the form. Then, as these little surges become longer and connect to one another, one becomes aware of the flow of chi through the Microcosmic Orbit. And finally, one learns to cycle chi more deliberately within the Microcosmic Orbit and then through the meridians of Macrocosmic Orbit lying within the limbs to produce various effects. Gradually after that, one begins to sense the greater chi field surrounding one's body. Then one can come to the realization that this greater field can be exploited by concentrating one's attention, first, on the strength of the field itself and, second, on one segment or one particular alignment of the field.

Concentrating attention on the strength of the whole-body field largely entails manipulating the power output of the Microcosmic Orbit. In a whole-body field at rest, the cascade of the field down and around the body exists equally in all directions and is constant in that it is always present. But its strength can be either amplified or dampened through breath manipulation. As pointed out earlier, this is effected not by the air of the breathing, per se, but by the abdominal muscles either squeezing or releasing pressure on the gut, where the chi is generated. A sharp exhale—or rapid compression of the abdominal muscles—pushes a surge of chi from the Conception Vessel into the base of the Governing Vessel, causing a greater force to fountain up the spine, accelerating the force of the whole-body field. A sharp inhale suddenly expands the abdominal muscles and sucks chi from the top of the Governing Vessel and down into the Conception Vessel, decelerating the force of the whole-body field. Effecting this sort of control is one objective of the Heng and Hah exercise mentioned in the chapter on breathing.

Placing attention on one segment of the field allows the practitioner to tap into and amplify the field's energy flow in that particular direction. To visualize this, imagine the energy of the whole-body field shooting up the core of your body and cascading down around your body. In a field at rest, this downward cascade is equal in all directions, but it is possible to concentrate your attention on only one half of the rotational planes of Push and Ward Off: either forward or backward. (Figure 6.31) This allows one to more forcefully rotate that portion of the whole-body field in that direction.

Concentrating on either the forward or backward segment of either the Push or Ward Off plane doesn't stop the cascade from going down elsewhere around you, but it gives mental precedence to the segment of the particular plane you concentrate on. This mental precedence creates not just a greater awareness of the field's rotation in the particular direction of concentration, but it changes the attention, which is passive, into intention, which is active. This intention can give the field greater density and impetus and create a temporarily stronger rotation in the direction of choice.

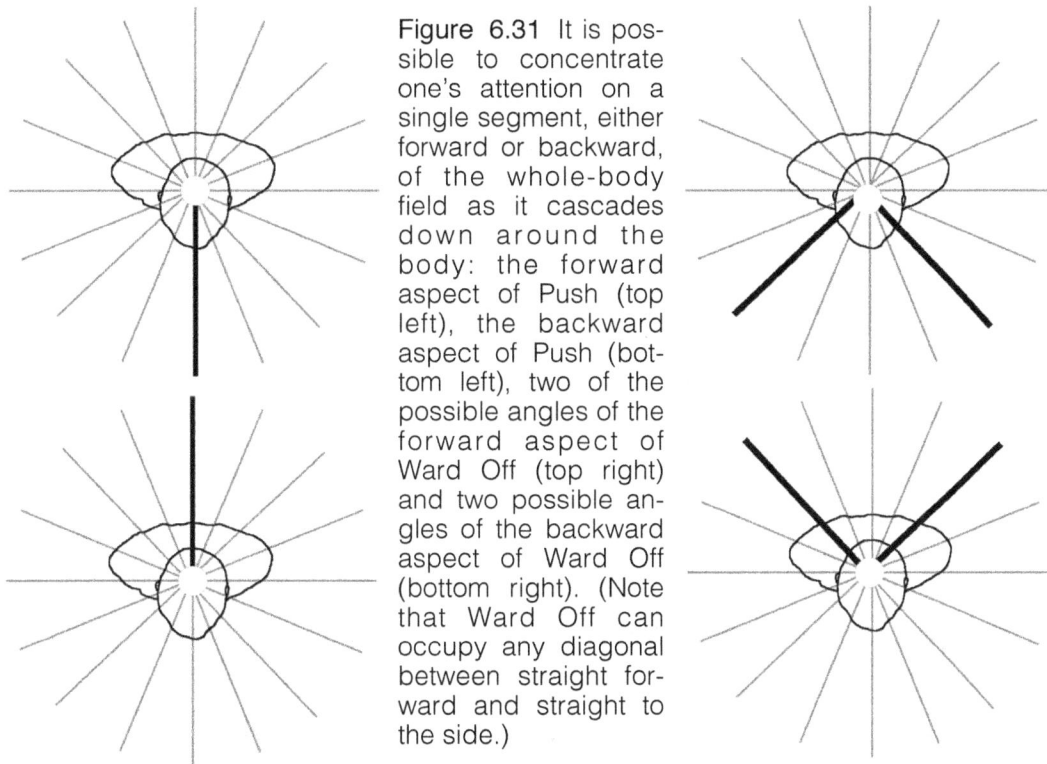

Figure 6.31 It is possible to concentrate one's attention on a single segment, either forward or backward, of the whole-body field as it cascades down around the body: the forward aspect of Push (top left), the backward aspect of Push (bottom left), two of the possible angles of the forward aspect of Ward Off (top right) and two possible angles of the backward aspect of Ward Off (bottom right). (Note that Ward Off can occupy any diagonal between straight forward and straight to the side.)

Because the whole-body field is created around the Microcosmic Orbit, the center of the field's rotation is half-way between the positive pole—the brain, the top tantien—and the negative pole—the enteric plexus, the lower tantien. (Figure 6.32) This places the center of rotation at about the level of your heart, which also is referred to as the middle tantien. The whole-body field's ultimate effective density and power depend on the strength of your energy's cyclical flow through the Microcosmic Orbit. It's important to repeat that the field does not stop operating in the areas of less concentration. It can't. One does not, for example, no longer have a left arm because one reaches out with the right hand to grasp a glass of water. Intention has simply caused the energy differential to grow greater in the right hand, motivating action in that direction. Likewise, the power output in a particular direction of the active biofield's rotation is increased and motivated by one's intention in that direction, assisted by the movements of the body, which physically help rotate the field in the same direction.

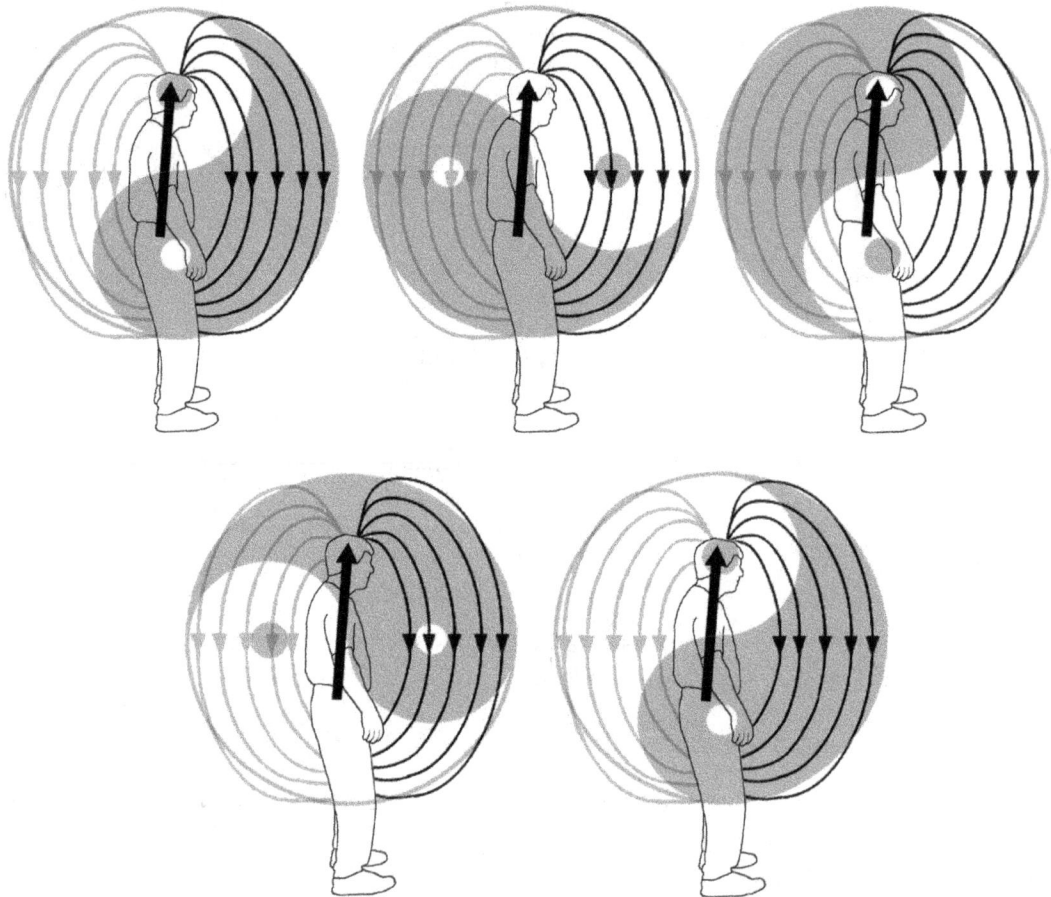

Figure 6.32 The cycling of the whole-body chi field can be affected along a given plane by one's intention, which can more strongly impel chi flow. Rolling Push energy forward is shown on this page, and rolling it backward is on the next page, and the reader can extrapolate for the various angles of Ward Off. The tai chi symbol indicates the direction in which the intention rotates the chi. The heavy arrow indicates the whole-body field's yang flow upward through the torso, the dark flow lines indicate the segment of the plane of the whole-body field where one pushes the field with one's intention, and the lighter flow lines indicate the reverse side of the plane, where one places no intention. Note that the energy and intention work together only during half of the cycle: the front half during the forward roll, and the back half during the backward roll.

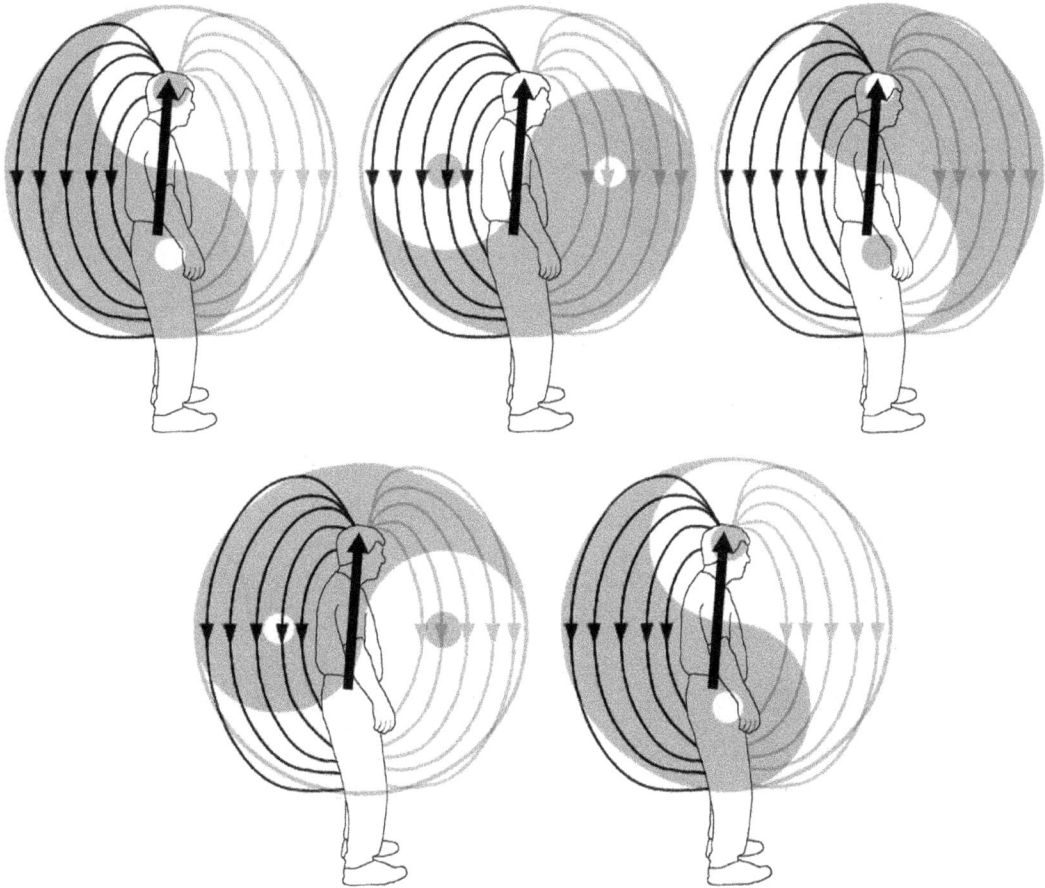

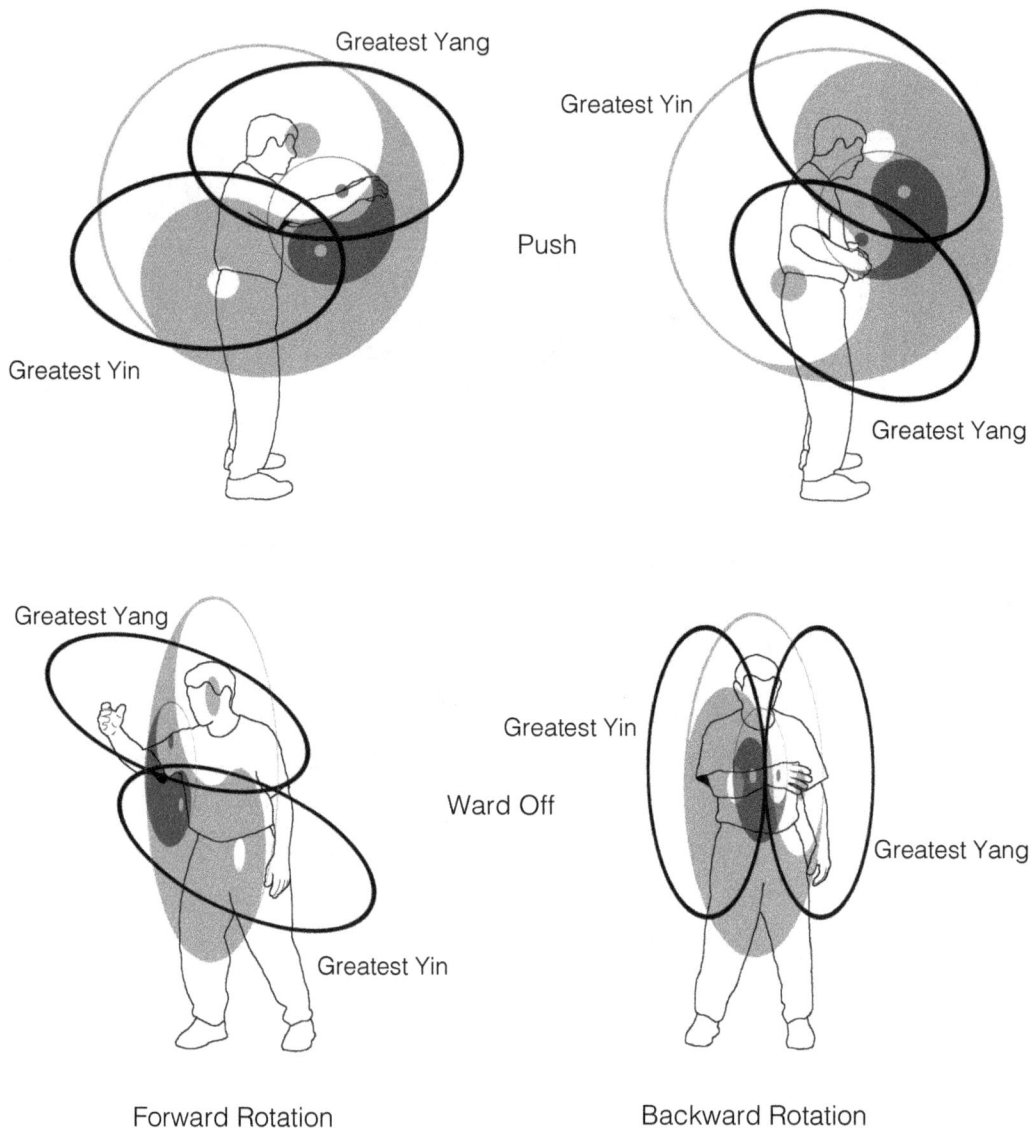

**Figure 6.33** When the rotation of the smaller, arm-created field works in sync with the larger, whole-body field, it amplifies the effects of the whole-body field where the two yang heads are in conjunction, and it reduces the effects of the whole-body field where the two Yin heads are in conjunction. If the two fields are not in conjunction, the offset will tend to nullify the effects of both fields, just as two equal sine waves in opposition cancel each other. This would created a case of energetic double-weighting.

We might object, since we recall from earlier that gravity deforms the passive field into an egg-shape, that such a shape in the active field would seem to prevent its ability to spin circularly. Gravitational deformation, however, holds true only for a field at rest—such as the passive field—or flowing perpendicularly to the gravitational field—such as that around a wire strung horizontally to the ground. The active portion of the whole-body field, on the other hand, is constantly cycling through and around the Microcosmic Orbit, and a spinning body is less affected by gravity than is a stationary one.

This can be seen in the workings of a gyroscope. When a gyroscope is at rest, its weight is unbalanced around the periphery of its wheel, and it will easily topple if you try to stand it on its foot. But once it is spinning, it effectively has exactly equal weight or force in all horizontal directions at once, so gravity affects it equally in all directions, allowing the gyroscope to actively stand on its end without falling over. In a similar manner, once one concentrates on spinning one's whole-body field in a single direction, it ceases to be as deformed by gravity. A human's active biofield is not as simple as a gyroscope, which operates in two dimensions—width and depth—to anchor itself in a third—height. It is a torus, which is a figure "generated by revolving a circle in three-dimensional space about an axis coplanar with the circle."[46] The basic torus shape is a donut-like ring that is energetically stable in all directions. Likewise, the human energy field is a torus that operates in three dimensions to anchor itself not just within the universal chi field, but perhaps in four dimensions. And none of this precludes the active portion of the whole-body field, because of its potentially large diameter, from embedding itself in the ground and within the Earth's magnetic field, just as the passive portion of the field does. In fact, the more powerful and dense the whole-body field, the more thoroughly it embeds.

Now that we've established the basic dynamics of the operation of the whole-body field and how Push and Ward Off interact with it, let's complexify the matter by adding the rotations, swirls, and currents that the arms can create within the whole-body field. We'll start with the simplest step of adding the effects of the arm movements of Push and Ward Off within a similar rolling of the whole-body field in the same direction. The key to this is that the rotation of the smaller, arm-created swirl must synchronize with the rotation of the larger field, in essence producing an aggregate effect that is more powerful than the rotation of either field alone. This is much like the way that two like sine waves can be combined to produce a higher peak amplitude—yang force—and a lower trough—yin force—than either sine wave alone.

Thus, the aggregate energetic effect of two yang energies moving together along a given plane produces amplification, while the aggregate effect of two yin energies moving together produces greater emptying. The yang effect can be either forward or backward, depending on the direction of rotation, and the yin effect is always on the opposite side of the rotation from the yang effect. (Figure 6.33) Trying to rotate the smaller circle in opposition to the larger circle's rotation would, of course, nullify the energy output. Like two sine waves in partial or complete opposition, it would create an energetic form of double-weighting. Try it—it's really difficult to do and it feels like you're accomplishing nothing in terms of both force and energy.

Now let's look at Roll Back. As noted before, unlike Push and Ward Off, which operate on vertical planes straight through the body's core, Roll Back operates on a horizontal plane around the body's core. We saw in an earlier chapter that Roll Back is the Cardinal Energy that, on a physical

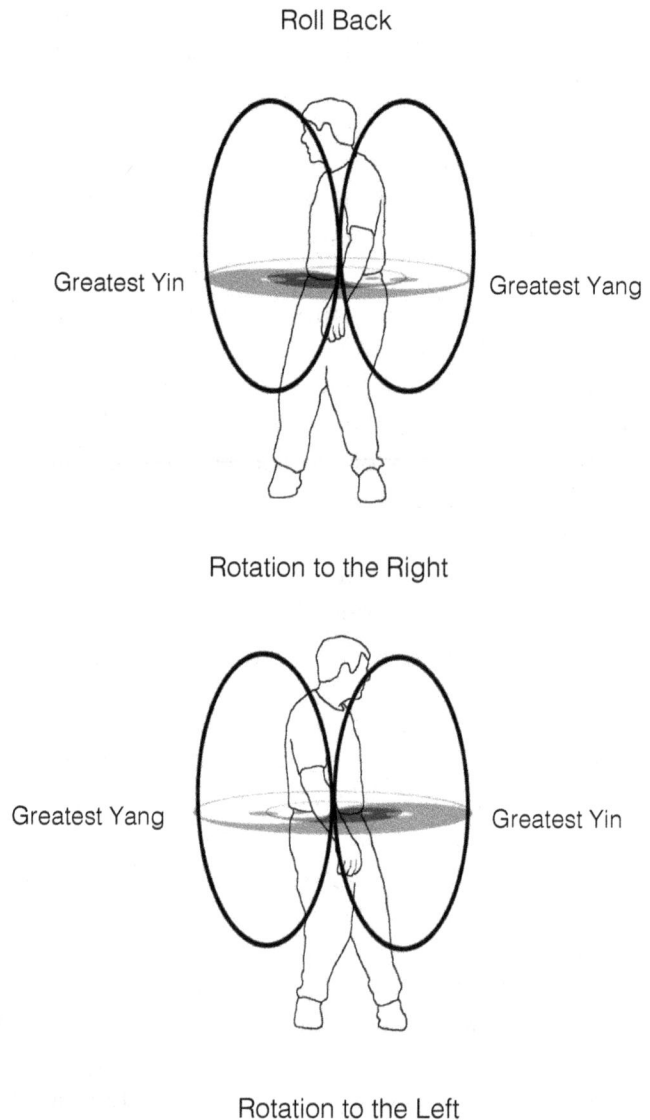

Roll Back

Greatest Yin

Greatest Yang

Rotation to the Right

Greatest Yang

Greatest Yin

Rotation to the Left

Figure 6.34 Using Roll Back to turn the whole-body field either to the right or to the left produces a diminishing energy effect in the direction of the turn.

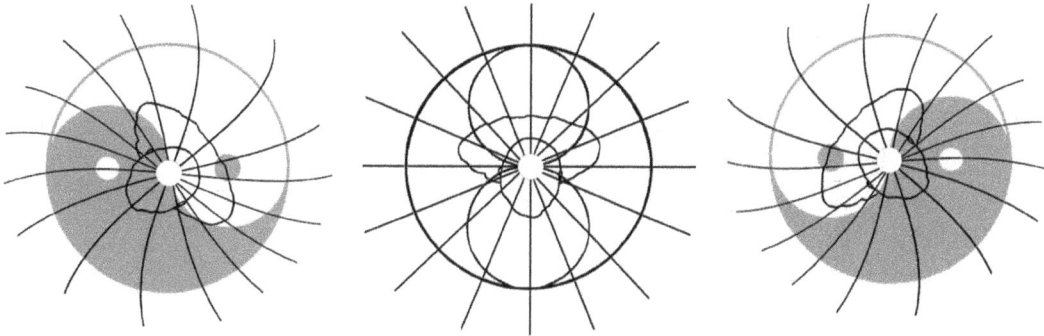

Figure 6.35 When one stands still (center) the energy of the whole-body field simply cascades downward around the body. But using Roll Back causes the whole-body field to twist with the turn. Turning to the right twists the field clockwise (left), and turning to the left twists the field counter-clockwise (right).

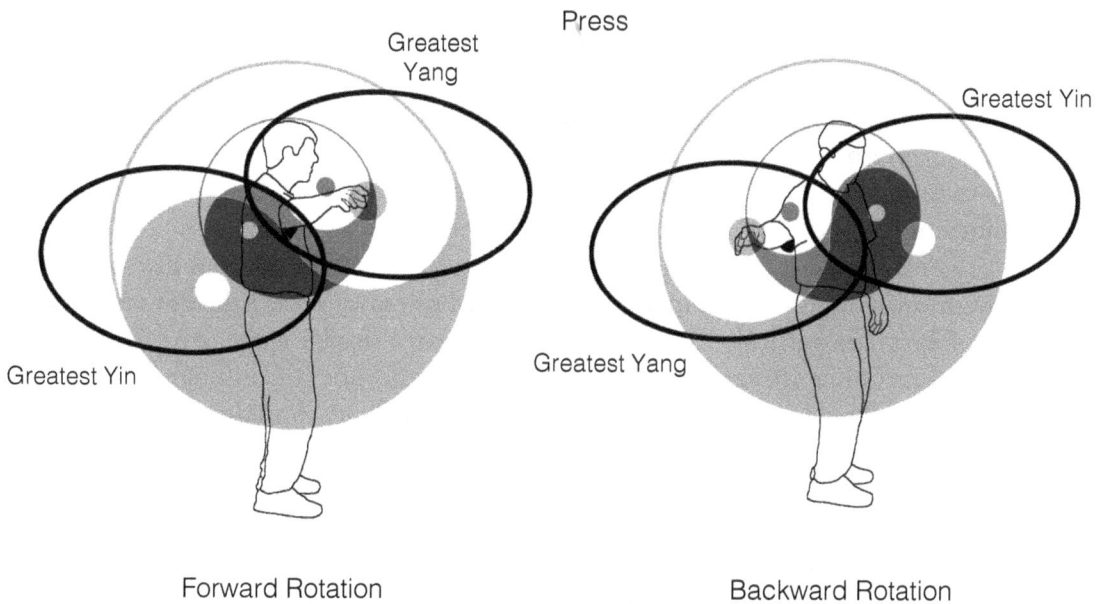

Press

Greatest Yang

Greatest Yin

Greatest Yin

Greatest Yang

Forward Rotation

Backward Rotation

Figure 6.36 As with the rotations of the other Cardinal Energy planes, the rotation of Press along a side axis has an aggregate effect on the movement's energy output.

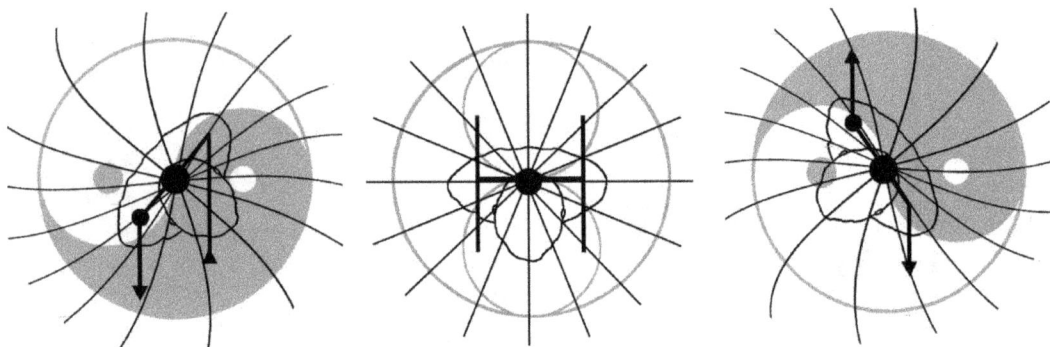

**Figure 6.37** Press twists the field in the direction of the yang force, whether forward (left) or backward (right), while the opposite side of the field is its yielding, yin side. The force-neutral position (center) embodies both possibilities.

level, gives Tai Chi's Ordinal Energies their coiling and twisting characteristics. But Roll Back also has an energetic effect on the whole-body field. As with Push and Ward Off, this effect is the creation of higher energy differentials, but unlike Push and Ward Off, where the energy differentials are in front of and behind you, Roll Back's differentials lie on the sides of the body, with the decrease or increase depending on the direction you turn. (Figure 6.34) A turn toward either direction decompresses the body's field in that direction and compresses it in the other. Roll Back's twisting, then, coils the whole-body field one way or another around Central Equilibrium. (Figure 6.35)

I've saved Press for last not only because it is quite interesting, but also because it is the most complex in its operation. As with Push and Ward Off, the rotational planes of Press are vertically oriented and can create a similar aggregate effect. (Figure 6.36), but unlike those energies, the Press planes do not run through the body's core. Instead, they run through the line of heel, hip, and shoulder, either on the right side or on the left. This leaves Press with a deficit because if Press were to rely solely on its vertical side plane of rotation, it could not generate much torque, but primarily forward or backward momentum.

We discussed these matters before when talking about Press on a physical level. And just as it hides a secret when operating physically, it also hides a secret on the energetic level in the way it employs Roll Back's horizontal plane. Unlike pure Roll Back, which swirls the whole-body field around the body's central vertical axis to divert incoming energy from an opponent to one side or the other around the periphery of the

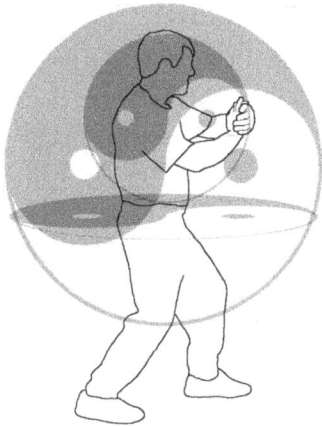

Figure 6.38 The aggregate effect of vertical and horizontal rotations gives Press its considerable power.

field, Press swirls the field to direct one's own energy either straight forward or straight backward through one side of the field or the other.

To see how this works, recall from the Press section in the chapter on the Thirteen Postures that, on a physical level, the key to Press is that the yin arm pulls, pushes, or swings in a direction perpendicular to the line of force of the yang arm. To Press forward, you pull the yin arm away from the yang arm, and to Press back- ward, you push the yin arm toward the yang arm. Both actions rotate the body around one of the two side vertical axes, one way or the other, and the movement thrusts one side forward and jerks the other side backward. (Figure 6.37)

Essentially, this transforms circular momentum into angular momentum—something we discussed in the section on power emission—and while this happens with Press on the purely physical level, it also occurs on the energetic level, with the twist around the axis automatically swirling the whole-body field. Again, the effect is much like that produced by a lever and fulcrum, with the pivot point of the right or left axis being the fulcrum. The more energy that is applied to the longer, yin end of the lever, the more pronounced and powerful the effect will be on the yang end. It's the same with the energy field, compounding Press's aggregate and often shocking release of force and energy, along with the fact that the rotation of the horizontal energy plane works in conjunction with the rotation of the vertical energy plane, making it possible to employ energetic torque and gravity assists from two complementary directions at once. (Figure 6.38)

In the expressions of all the rotational fields of the Cardinal Energies, combining the physical movements of the limbs with the movement of both the active chi field and the currents created within it by the limbs doesn't just produce a strengthening of the active field in the yang direction and a weakening of the field in the yin direction. As with combining the peaks and troughs of two like sine waves to create a higher amplitude, it actually physically deforms the larger field, enlarging it in the yang direction and diminishing it in the yin direction. This also takes us back to the idea that flattening the pure circles of the Cardinal Energies into ovals can produce a more pronounced effect in both the yang and yin directions. So, if one flattens the pure Cardinal Energy circles created by the arms into ovals, the arms' fields and the body's movements would create a similarly pronounced bulge in the whole-body field.

Obviously it would be difficult, if not impossible—and certainly pedantic—to attempt to enumerate all the possible energy swirls that Tai Chi's arm movements can create in the whole-body field. In any case, I'm not enough of an artist to draw them all. But hopefully these basic examples will encourage the reader to experiment and discover the varieties on his or her own.

> In the vertical scheme of the human body, the focal points are three in number: the brain, the heart and the sexual organs. But the central point is the heart, and in consequence it comes to partake of the meanings of the other two ... for all centers are symbols of the wheel of phenomena rotating around the Aristotelian 'unmoved mover.'
>
> —J. E. Cirlot[45]

# Peng and Fa Jin

**Now let's look** at Peng. By this I mean the force behind Tai Chi's power, not the word Peng as a name for Ward Off. As with other topics tackled in this book, I did a fair amount of research on Peng to see how it is defined by various Tai Chi experts. Most of them agree that Peng is the force behind Tai Chi's power, but beyond that, I found a lot of talk that skirts a solid definition, despite articles like, "Peng Jin Explained," which did not explain anything, and "On Internal Power," which had a lot to say about what Peng isn't. So, as with many Tai Chi concepts and principles, I was forced to experiment and come up with my own definition. I'll explain what I think Peng is, and that will lead to a discussion of fa jin and a few of the ways it manifests. From there, in the next section, I'll dissect a very specific and rather complex expression of fa jin: the floating punch.

Earlier, I described the sensation of being startled, say, by a loud sound, in which it seems as if a body-shaped force inside you moves suddenly, and the body responds by jerking back into alignment with this inner body. This inner body is your chi body—the portion of your whole-body field that you can directly sense because it lies within the boundaries of your skin. This is not to say that the chi field is limited to the boundaries of the flesh. It isn't, and it can be either small or large, as we've seen. We've all known people who lack vitality. These are folks whose chi field is weak and whose energy does not seem to completely fill them. And we've also met other people who radiate vitality. They are the ones whose fields are strong and whose chi bodies seem to swell beyond their skin.

Being startled and having your chi body jerk in response is a case of your nervous

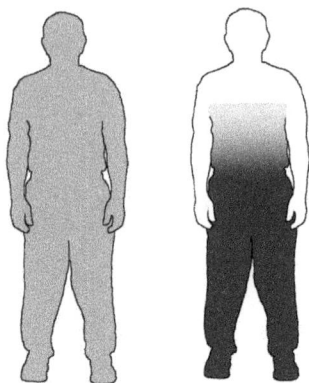

Figure 6.40 Left, an unre-
fined chi body diffusely
fills the physical body.
Right, a refined chi body
is sunken and condensed
into the lower part of the
physical body.

system flaring up in a sudden, random, and undirect-
ed avoidance response to abrupt external stress, causing a similar flare up in your bioelectromagnetic field.
This causes a slight gap before your flesh and your
chi body resynchronize with a snap. Tai Chi, on the
other hand, gives one the tools to deliberately manipulate the chi field, and thus, the chi body. It is a
process of intentionally activating the chi body in
ways that cause it to purposefully coalesce and to rebound and surge inside the body in a controlled
manner that can send a wave or wash of energy into
specific areas, such as a shoulder or limb.

So, here's my definition: To deliberately motivate
the chi body within the physical body—and thus to
appropriately manipulate the biofield as a whole—is
to Peng. As we've learned in previous chapters, all
Tai Chi movements enable one to motivate and direct one's chi within the body and limbs and to rotate the active chi field in conjunction with the
body's physical movements. And as I also stated previously, this chi body should not
completely fill the body from sole to crown but should be sunken into the lower abdomen. (Figure 6.40) This sinking is one aspect of the Tai Chi concept called Sung
(also spelled Song). Sung is a fairly complex activity that relies on several aspects:

1.) A proper upright body alignment helps prevent the chi from accumulating in the chest, shoulders, and arms and allows it to sink
downward. This includes relaxing the shoulders and dropping the
elbows as well as a slightly sunken stance, with the knees flexed, the
back straight, and the buttocks tucked in, causing a sensation as if
one is sitting on a three-legged stool, two of whose legs are the
body's own legs and the third of which is an invisible extension of
the spine, or, Central Equilibrium.

2.) A firm foundation gives one stability and aids in rooting one's energy. This begins at the bottom and works its way up, and the first
task is to learn to relax the soles of the feet to allow them to make
full and solid contact with the ground. The lower legs must then be

aligned properly with the feet to take advantage of the ankles' full range of motion while protecting the ankles—two of the most vulnerable joints of the body—from injury. Next, one must correctly position the thighs to accomplish the same tasks for the knees—another set of relatively weak joints. This solid foundation allows the chi to flow properly through the lower channels of the Nine-Channel Pearl, and it also creates a stable bowl of the pelvis, into which you sit your upper body—elastically connected and responsive to your lower body but independently relaxed. A long term benefit is the retention of stability and balance into old age.

3.) Relaxation of joints and unnecessary muscular tension above the waist releases blockages and tension that retard chi flow in the upper body and blanket the sensitivity required to feel the chi, both as flow and as field. Relaxation, along with an upright body posture, allows and assists the chi body to drain downward, out of the head and chest and into the lower parts of the body. The result is a condition of muscular vitality and strength below the waist and of loose elasticity above the waist in which movement is accomplished by the fasciae and tendons instead of muscle—"heavy on bottom, light on top."

4.) Abdominal breathing calms, regularizes, and deepens the breath, helping ease upper-body tension. It also causes the breathing muscles to press downward on the viscera, generating a more powerful bioelectromagnetic force and increasing the power of the engine that pushes the chi through the Microcosmic and Macrocosmic Orbits. This assists also in creating the rolling ball of energy in the tantien.

On the level of physiological manipulation of chi energy, Peng is actually rolling the active field in whatever direction you need to, but from the inside, the sensation feels very much like "sloshing" the chi body around inside the physical body. Remember, the "substance" of the biofield is fluid, even if it is tenuous, and it is elastically connected to the physical body. This sloshing cannot be accomplished if the chi body diffusely fills the entire body from the sole to crown. The chi body must be sunken into the abdomen in part to give it greater heft for sloshing and in part to allow space for the condensed chi body to slosh into. After all, one cannot have action—yang—without space in which the action can occur—yin.

Let's look a little more closely at this sloshing by using several concrete examples. The basic Shoulder Strike is a fairly straightforward kind of Peng that involves sloshing the chi body only within the torso and shoulder. (Figure 6.41) Movements like Brush Knee Twist Step and Slant Flying are more complex examples of Peng because they involve sloshing the chi body not just within the torso, but into a limb. This necessitates manipulation of the flow into the legs and arms by constricting the appropriate muscles surrounding the sacral and brachial plexes, as discussed previously in relation to chi flow into the limbs. You can extrapolate the sloshing of the chi body—forward, backward, or to either side—to many other

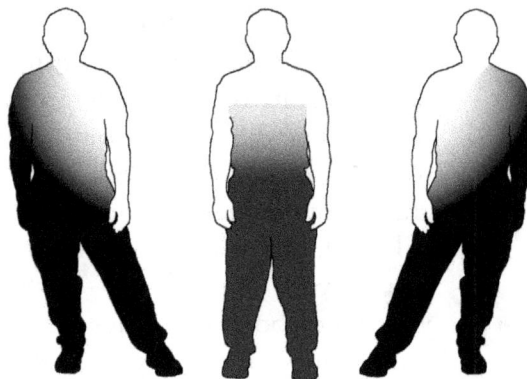

Figure 6.41 Peng is the action of moving the sunken chi body around inside the physical body. It is much like sloshing liquid around inside a container.

movements, such as Press and Ward Off, and movements where the Peng force is directed straight into a body part can be considered yang Peng.

But every movement has its yin and yang aspect in combination, and the yin aspect can be seen specifically as the sucking energy of the void vacated by the sloshing. A portion of the Grasping Bird's Tail sequence from the form I do begins by sloshing backward to draw in an opponent and then sloshing forward to expel him. (Figure 6.42) Just as one can use mind-intent to isolate and manipulate one segment of the whole-body field, as described in the previous section, mind-intent can focus on and control the force and quality of the part of the sloshing—yang or yin—on which you place your attention, as well as the direction of the sloshing. The yang side of a slosh produces a repelling force, while the yin side produces an inward-drawing force. In this respect, the effects are similar to the energies created by waves at a beach. A wave washing into shore produces force, while a retreating wave creates an undertow.

Forward and backward sloshing are characteristic of the Cardinal Energies of Ward Off, Press, and Push, but Roll Back adds a twisting dimension, causing the chi body to swirl in a circular manner. This swirling is characteristic of the Ordinal Energies, where the chi body whips outward in a spinning motion or inward into a vortex. The former releases yang energy, as can be seen, for example, in Elbow

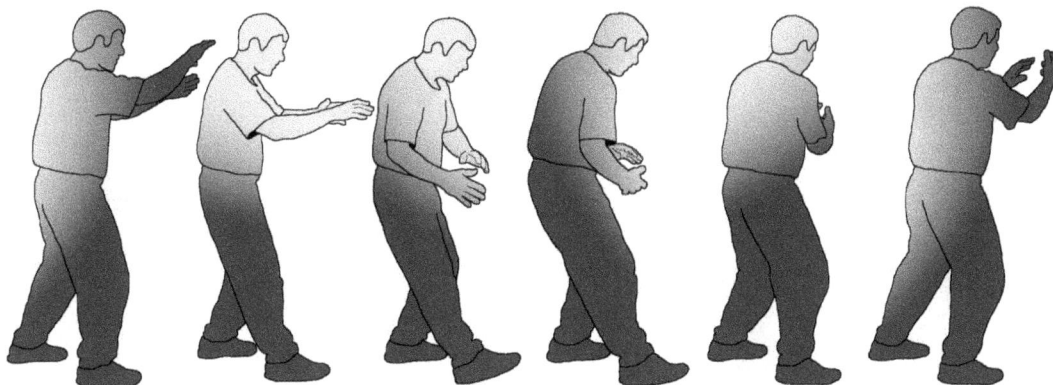

Figure 6.42 Grasping Bird's Tail (Ward Off) showing Peng's sloshing effect.

Strike, and the latter produces yin energy, as can be seen in some usages of Pull/ Pluck. In practice, both actually work together—one cannot have yang without yin, and vice versa. Elbow Strike, for example, is frequently the same movement as Pull/ Pluck, the difference being the direction in which mind-intent focuses the action. In fact, almost all Tai Chi movements embody a sloshing that is both directional and twisting—again, a combination of linear force and torque. Figure 6.43 shows several common Tai Chi postures filled with directed Peng. These examples are, of course, very basic and meant to illustrate the point. The reader will have to use his or her imagination and personal sensations to discover all the possible permutations possible within the various Tai Chi postures.

One can see from these examples that the internal sloshing of the chi body— Peng, an energy manipulation—is intimately linked to Tai Chi's whipping, folding and unfolding, and torquing—the physical movements of leading the energy through the Nine-Channel Pearl in various ways and directions. But the reverse is not true: One can use a whipping or pulling movement that is not filled with Peng but that relies solely on muscular force. A whipping or pulling that is empty of Peng is external martial arts, while these same movements, filled with Peng, are Tai Chi. In other words, physical whipping and pulling are not Peng, they only provide the proper scaf- fold—body alignments and movements—to support Peng and allow its expression.

Similarly, Peng is not fa jin. One can Peng without doing fa jin—one can slosh but not cause the sloshing to produce fa jin force—but one cannot produce fa jin force without sloshing the chi body to create Peng. Peng is deliberate movement of

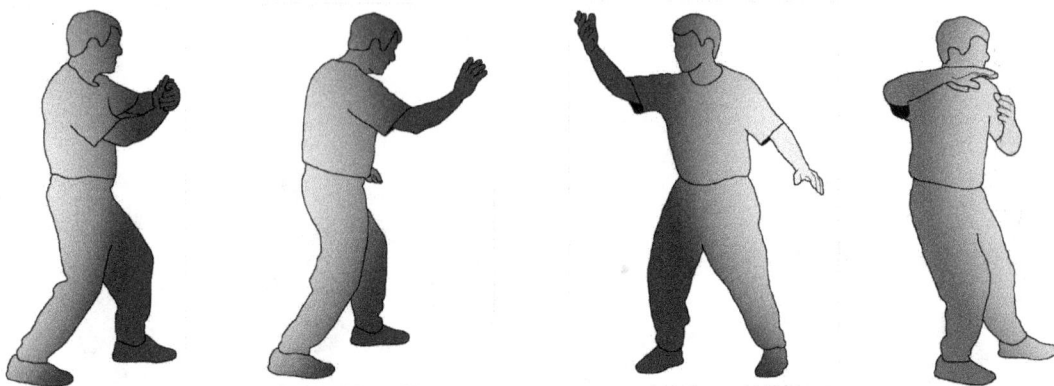

Figure 6.43 Peng is manifested in most Tai Chi movements. These are just a few examples: (left to right) Press, Brush Knee Twist Step, Slant Flying, and Elbow Strike.

the chi body into a receiving body part, while fa jin entails specific manipulations of Peng energy that causes it to have more power for direct external utility. In order for Peng energy to create fa jin, one must use mind intent to rapidly and forcefully surge the chi body into or out of appropriate body parts and momentarily and firmly coalesce it at a focal point. The more forcefully one surges, coalesces, and focuses the energy, the more powerful the fa jin. Again, to liken this to waves at the beach, there can be the gentle lapping of waves against the shore—Peng alone—or huge, pounding waves—highly impelled Peng, or, fa jin. The water is the same and the action is the same; the difference is the power with which the water is moved.

Now, think of a forceful wave surging into an ever-narrowing cove. The force and energy of the wave would then be focused into the apex of the cove and would impart great power when it rushes into that point. The same thing happens in fa jin when the Peng energy is surged forcefully into an ever-narrowing limb. But of course, the body's biofield is not confined within the boundaries of the flesh, so when you Peng, you might feel the force of the chi field shift only inside of your skin, but it also is similarly impelled in the space outside of your body—remember, energy fields merge before bodies collide.

But the force with which the Peng energy is moved isn't the whole story. We also have to add Tai Chi's special dynamics, in particular, the way one can flatten the circles of the pure Cardinal Energies into ovals to create a more powerful manifestation of force and chi, as described previously. The amount of the combined physical force and chi power is controlled by how much we flatten the Cardinal Energy ovals. And even this isn't enough. We also have to whip the energy around and through the recurves of the two tai chi symbol fish and then bring it up short, as described in the section on power emission.

Tactically, Tai Chi utilizes conscious actions, which tend to be complex, purposeful, and slow, but through repetitive training in movement patterns and control of internal energies, these conscious actions can be internalized to such a degree that they can operate in the context of the much faster and unconscious reaction process. In this way, Tai Chi combines complexity and purpose with speed and sensitivity to deliver physical force and energetic power tied to rapidly circulating torque on two cooperating and tightly focused planes.

> When a person trained in Chi development has achieved Small Circulation and Grand Circulation, he can use the Chi generated at the Dan Tien. The energy passes through the Sea Bottom cavity and is led to the feet, and it is also led up the spine and out to the hands. When Chi from the Dan Tien is used to support the tendons, the Jing can reach a high level.
>
> —Yang Jwing-Ming[47]

# The Floating Punch

**The internal-style** Tai Chi punch—more properly referred to as the "floating punch"—warrants special attention due to the more complex way in which it operates when compared to the average, external-style punch. Please understand that in what follows I'm not saying that an external-style punch can't be fast and powerful and have devastating effects. As with any martial art, it's not the style that counts, but the expertise of the martial artist. I'm simply trying to parse the differences between it and the floating punch that, I think, demonstrate that the floating punch has distinct advantages.

Even though the external-style punch and the floating punch are quite different in structure, they do have a few similarities. The two have vaguely similar physical motions when looked at from the outside, and they certainly have the similar goal of using the fist to inflict damage on an opponent. The most important similarity, though, is the way one aligns the forearm, wrist, and fist. No matter what kind of punch you use, these alignments are critical, first, to effectively transmit the power of the punch down the arm and into the fist and, second, to protect the wrist and fingers from being damaged upon impact. In all cases, the surface of the outside of the forearm, the back of the wrist, and the back of the hand should all line up. (Figure 6.44) This straight line allows the force of the punch to travel straight down the bones of the forearm, through the wrist, and into the knuckles, and it also prevents the wrist from bending forward or backward upon impact, either of which could sprain or break it.

In both the external-style punch and the floating punch, one could simply thrust the fist straight forward, which would mean that the prominent knuckle of the middle finger would be foremost. This might work well in some instances, such

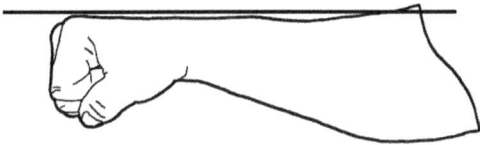

Figure 6.44 When punching, straight arm alignments properly transmit the force and protect the wrist.

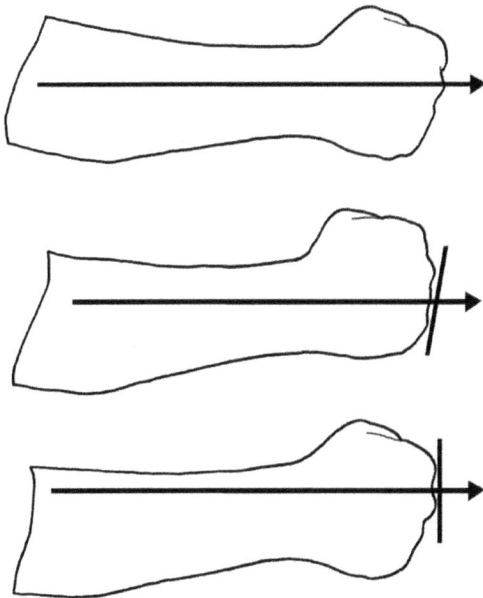

Figure 6.45 A straight fist (top) can leave the middle knuckle vulnerable to injury. Angling the fist up (middle) presents a flat surface with few protrusions for striking hard areas, and angling the fist down (bottom) presents a sharper surface for striking softer areas.

as abdominal punches, but it leaves the middle knuckle vulnerable to fracture on impact against bony areas. So, in both styles of punches, there are two alternatives in which one twists the fist upward or downward on the wrist to present two very different striking surfaces that not only can help prevent breaking the middle knuckle, but can use selective targeting to maximize the value of the punch. (Figure 6.45) Note that this twisting is lateral to the straight line outlined above and does not bend the wrist forward or backward. Twisting the fist upward presents a surface consisting of the last three knuckles. This is a relatively flat surface that distributes the force of the blow across the line of the three knuckles, and it is useful for striking hard, flat surfaces that might damage the middle knuckle if it is used alone, such as the jaw bone, plane of the cheek, chest, or rib cage.

Twisting the fist downward on the wrist presents a striking surface consisting of the first two knuckles. This is a sharper surface and thus has greater penetrating power, but it allows the force of the impact to be distributed between the first two knuckles instead of being taken mostly by the middle knuckle. It is more useful for striking softer areas, such as the gut, the kidneys, muscles, and cavities. A cavity is an indention between muscles or between bones and muscle.

An example of the former is the indentation between the bicep and tricep on the inside of the upper arm, and an example of the latter is the solar plexus. (Figure 6.46) Quite often, bundles of nerves and their associated meridians lie within cavities, and they can be hurt or damaged by a penetrating strike. In kung fu lingo, this is called "sealing the cavity," and the re-

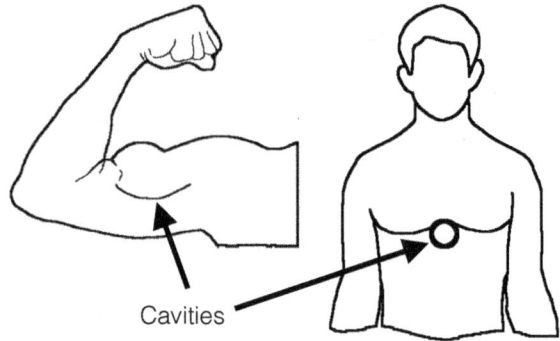

Figure 6.46 Two examples of cavities: the one between the bicep and tricep (left) and the solar plexus, just below the sternum (right).

sult can be not only severe pain, but also temporary paralysis of the body parts associated with the nerves and meridians in the cavity. Sealing the cavity between the bicep and tricep will paralyze the arm. A penetrating but light strike to the solar plexus will cause the victim to have difficulty in breathing, while a very powerful strike there could so paralyze the nerves that the victim will be unable to breathe at all.

Before we move on to the differences between the external-style and floating punches, let's look a little more closely at some interesting aspects of the two ways outlined above to present the fist. If you think back on the passages in the section on Pull/Pluck, you'll recall that Pluck, which is performed above the waist, uses the thumb and first two fingers, while Pull, which is performed below the waist, uses the last three fingers. We also recall that the thumb, first finger, and part of the middle finger, are activated by one set of nerves that run from the inside of the shoulder to the fingertips through the top inside of the arm, while the pinky, ring finger, and part of the middle finger are activated by a second set of nerves that run from the fingertips to the bottom outside of the shoulder through the outside of the arm. These nerves are contiguous with the meridians that carry chi: in the case of the former set, from the brachial plexus to the hand, and in the case of the latter set, from the hand back into the brachial plexus. And from the section on fasciae, we know that Pull uses the fasciae on the bottom inside of the arm, while Pluck uses the fasciae on the upper outside of the arm.

In a like manner, the two alternate ways to present the fist have a different orientation with regard to structures inside the forearm, namely, the two bones there: the ulna and the radius. Of these, the ulna is the heavier and runs through the bottom part of the forearm, while the radius is the lighter and runs though the top of the forearm. Angling the wrist downward to present the first two knuckles will cause the line of force from elbow to knuckles to use the radius as its axis of thrust, and angling the wrist upward to present the last three knuckles will cause the force to use the ulna as its axis of thrust. If you experiment with both angles, you can feel that the energy of each originates in a different part of the shoulder: the top outside of the shoulder when using the first two knuckles, and the bottom inside of the shoulder when using the last three knuckles. I'm not sure that this means that each angle can be strictly associated with either the outbound meridians for the first two knuckles or the inbound ones for the last three knuckles, but that's a strong possibility. Certainly the appropriate fasciae are involved, and most likely, associated nerves, meridians, and fasciae, as well as the bones, all operate in conjunction during floating punches.

Moving on: While some elements of an external-style punch and the floating punch overlap, the differences between the two types of punches are more pronounced than are the similarities. When one punches, there are several things to consider: how the punching power is generated, how the punch is delivered, how the muscles of the arm and hand work together to make the fist, and how the muscles control the physical force and chi energy flowing through the arm to further empower the punch. All of these aspects affect the force, power, and speed of the punch, and in each case, the floating punch is executed in a radically different way than is the external-style punch.

We'll begin with the way punching power is generated. While some external-style experts and boxers can and do generate whole-body power, most external-style punching power is generated primarily in the shoulder and arm, with a number of muscles in the torso and back also coming into play. The power of such a punch is limited by two factors: the strength of the muscles in the torso and arm throwing the punch and the weight of the body behind the punch. Because the external-style punch primarily uses the muscles of the upper body, it engages only the static weight of the body itself—the weight of the body as registered on a scale. A heavy-weight boxer, for example, can throw a more powerful punch than can a light-weight boxer at the same basic skill level simply because he has more strength and weight behind the punch.

We can contrast this with the way the floating punch is generated. I discussed the dynamics of this at some length in earlier chapters, showing that the floating punch is a variety of Press because all the force and energy are generated and expressed around one of the side axes and along a single side of the body. In short, the

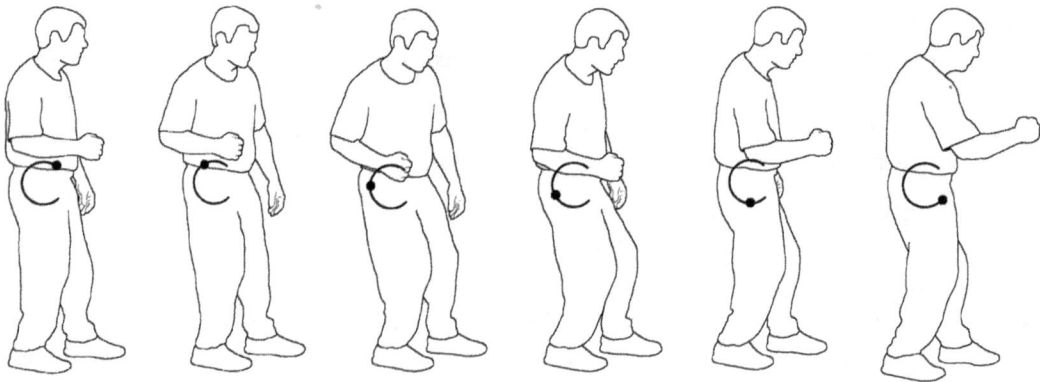

**Figure 6.47** The fist of the floating punch is impelled by a C-shaped circling of the hips. Circling from top to bottom is shown here, but the circling can go from bottom to top for head-high punches and some other Press movements, such as Brush Knee Twist Step.

power of a floating punch is not generated in the shoulder and arm but comes, instead, from two factors. The first is vertically circling the hip on the same side as the striking arm in a C-shape to generate linear force along the vertical Press plane. For punching, this circling is always backward and then forward around the C, but it can circle either from the top to the bottom or from the bottom to the top. Each one produces a different kind of punch.

One would tend to roll the C from top to bottom for a gut punch. (Figure 6.47) Conversely, one would tend to roll the C from bottom to top for an upper-body punch. Brush Knee Twist Step, though usually employing an open palm instead of a fist, is an example of this. But this breakdown doesn't always hold true enough to form a rule. An uppercut, for example, rolls the C from top to bottom, yet the target can be the head. So the rule is simply to roll the C in the proper direction for the type of punch you wish to execute. The C is, of course, "the curved," or a parabolic arc, and the punching arm is "the straight," or the tangent flung outward from the parabolic arc. Thus, a punch is a perfect example of "seeking the straight in the curved." Also, recall the driving wheel of a locomotive.

In essence, rolling the C vertically in either direction causes one to go into a brief and controlled free fall toward the bottom of the C. Various Tai Chi exponents refer to this action as "sinking," "sitting," or "settling"—terms I've mentioned before. I like the last term best because settling implies a curving back and forth

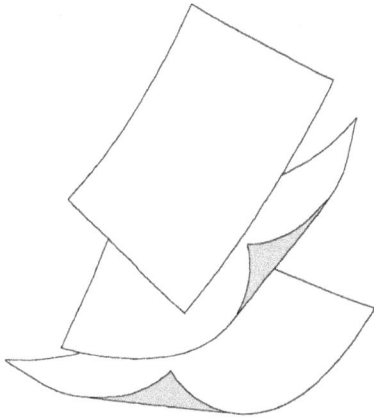

Figure 6.48 A falling piece of paper settles, rather than falls straight down.

motion rather than a simple dropping downward. Think of a leaf, a feather, or a piece of paper settling to the floor. (Figure 6.48) A highly obvious example of whole-body settling is Snake Creeps Down, in which one sinks backward and downward, then comes out of that in a forceful, upward arcing curve into Golden Cock Stands on One Leg. The settling and upthrust of Beating Tiger is another good example. (Figure 6.49)

The settling done in punching is exactly the same but is executed in a very much tighter scope and only around one hip instead of with the whole body. But the body isn't perfectly weightless during the punch's brief and controlled free fall because Earth's gravity continually causes it to accelerate—at least for the short distance you circle downward through the C. You can tap into this acceleration to create a seed of momentum that can then sprout into a forceful surge out of the free fall. The momentum is further accelerated by the sudden, piston-like thrust of the leg muscles, which push the body, either forward from the bottom through the downward curve or upward and forward through the upward curve. This curving motion takes advantage of

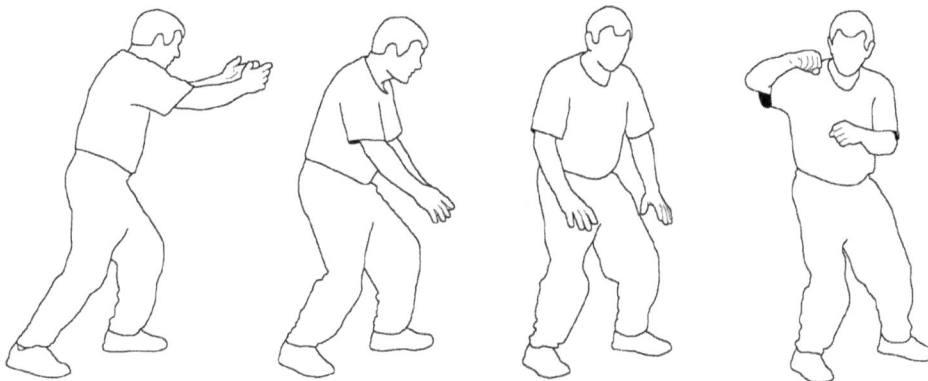

Figure 6.49 Whole-body settling in Beating Tiger.

the continuous momentum of the controlled free fall to eliminate the inertia that might occur if one were to simply sink or sit straight down then push upward. It's an example of an old friend from an earlier chapter: the gravity assist.

Furthermore, the force and energy imparted by settling or sinking don't just move straight down the leg then straight back up but spiral in both directions due to the torque imparted by the twisting of the waist and the corkscrew structure of the fasciae in the legs. We talked a little about this in a previous section of this chapter. The downward spiral is given impetus by the free fall, and the energy is loaded into the elastic structures of the superficial back, superficial front, deep front, and spiral fascial lines. The upward spiral is propelled by the combination of a gravity assist powered by a muscular surge from the leg, releasing the energy compressed in the fascial lines, and a surge of chi energy in the form of Peng. The direction you spiral the force and energy down the leg and then back up depends on the direction you rotate the C: clockwise when rotating back, down, and forward, counterclockwise when rotating back, up, and forward. Interestingly, the energy of this spiraling does not spiral down to the foot, stop, then spiral upward. Because of its circularity, it can change direction in the sole of the foot just like Chan-ssu Chin can change direction without a pause through the tai chi symbol's recurved line and, just as the tai chi symbol rotating through the diagram of the Golden Spiral, can spiral inward to an infinitely small point then spiral outward without pause. The energy never stops moving, and in fact, this spiraling effect in the energetic leg is present in any expression of fa jin, not just in the floating punch, except where fa jin is expressed in Push, which can't take advantage of transverse torque.

In punching, these combined actions not only put the entire body weight behind the punch and dramatically add to that weight by the power of the gravity assist, it gives the ability to punch with a longer chain of muscles—foot through leg and torso to arm and fist—rather than just from torso to arm and fist. (Figure 6.50) Further, you are creating an unbroken line of strength and energy from the ground to your fist. This means that, in a sense, that the floating punch backs up its power not only with gravity-assisted, amplified body weight, but also the weight and solidity of the Earth itself, while the external-style punch is backed up only by the weight and solidity of the puncher's body. The amplified body weight thus produced can lend a light-weight the punching power of a heavy-weight—and more.

The power of the floating punch is further amplified by the torque imparted by twisting the waist and hips. Again, we've looked at this aspect in previous discussions of Press, so we can recognize the secondary, waist-generated horizontal plane of moment

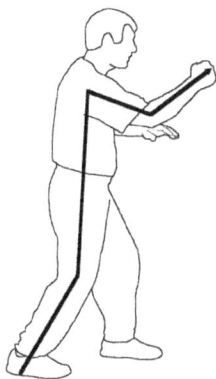

Figure 6.50 The floating punch produces power over a distance of six or seven feet.

that combines its own torquing gravity assist with the one generated by the hip on the vertical plane. The combined forces of the vertically and horizontally generated energies are focused together on a single spot, which, again, is lined up, along the vertical plane, directly into the ground. This combination not only exponentially increases the power of the punch, it also directly affects how the punch is delivered.

Some readers might object here that one can stand in an evenly weighted stance and rotate around the spine to punch, but if you experiment with that movement, you will see that this is not possible to accomplish without disengaging the upper body from the lower, resulting in a punch that issues strictly from the upper body, not the whole body—certainly not the Tai Chi way. To make the punch truly a floating punch, you must shift your weight from one leg to the other, which allows torque to be created. In fact, the very act of twisting the waist entails a stance that is not evenly weighted to some degree because to twist, you have to push off of one leg or the other, which automatically creates a yin/yang state in the legs—eliminating double-weighting.

If the hips do not lend torque to the movement, the pushing, yang leg cannot properly add its force to the punch, and the waist cannot transfer that force to the torso and arms. In this case, all the linear force, instead of coming up from the feet, through the body, and out the arm, is trapped in the chest and shoulders and can only be expressed from there. This makes a punch only as powerful as the torso, shoulders, and arms—an external-style punch. Further, this emphasis on the upper body creates a top-heavy situation in the puncher that can be exploited.

Because an external-style punch is thrown from the torso, shoulder, and arm, in order for it to develop sufficient energy to inflict damage, it must have a relatively long "throw"—the distance from the punch's launch to its impact point—to build sufficient momentum to do its work. In an external-style punch, this is accomplished by drawing the arm back to some degree or another, then thrusting it forward. Even the short-range jab requires this backward/forward action, and in a sense, the jab proves the point, for it is a relatively weak punch precisely because its draw and throw are extremely short.

The floating punch, on the other hand, does not require a similar pulling back of the striking arm because its draw relies on the vertical circling of the hip in conjunction with the torquing action of the waist. This means that the striking fist can virtually float in space while the hips and waist rotate. The arm becomes actively engaged and moves with those rotations only when the vertical and horizontal forces align in conjunction at, or close to, the punch's point of focus. In other words, the draw of the Tai Chi punch is not a pulling back of the striking arm but a double circling of the hip and waist that launches the punch forward without a significant spacial draw-back of the arm and with little throw. Such a punch has been called Tai Chi's one-foot punch because, in that one-foot distance of punching movement, virtually all of the movement and power of the legs, waist, torso, and punching arm are gathered together behind one short but powerful forward thrust.

The briefer and more controlled the free fall is, the tighter the C becomes and, thus, the shorter the distance the fist has to travel to its target, so it can impact very quickly and at very close distances yet retain its full power. Some martial artists, most notably Bruce Lee, have refined the combined vertical circling of the hip and the horizontal torquing of the waist to such a degree that they can position all the elements of force behind the punch in a distance of as little as an inch. Theoretically, if a superior Tai Chi expert can touch you, he can turn that touch into a strike backed by full-body power. This is, of course, one element of fa jin, and it can be accomplished with just about any part of the body, not just the fist.

Another aspect regarding speed is the length of time it takes to draw the punch. The draw and launch of the external-style punch requires that the fist be drawn back a certain distance, say, fifteen inches. Then it must decelerate to a dead stop before it can be launched forward. This dead stop might last only a fraction of a second, but after that, the muscles of the shoulder and arm have to break the momentary inertia created by that split second of stillness before they can accelerate the fist forward. Then, the forward movement of the fist adds another, say, twenty-four inches of traveling distance to impact. All of this takes time, and even worse, some of the energy of the movement—namely the draw back, deceleration, breaking the inertia, and reacceleration of the fist—is essentially wasted.

The circular launch of the floating punch can give it a traveling distance of a foot or less without a time- and energy-consuming draw back. But even though the actual draw of the floating punch is negligible, the circularity of the vertical wind-up of the rotating hip and the body's alignments from ground to fist gives it a far greater virtual length—a distance that, in practical terms, goes all the way down to the sole of the foot of the pistoning leg. This gives the virtual draw of the floating punch a distance of five or six feet to power its actual launch distance of one foot or less. Even better, much of this launch is impelled by the leg, which contains the body's most powerful muscles, backed by the solidity of the ground. Remember, the leg is the body's analog to the Saturn rocket's main booster stage.

And the beauty of the floating punch is that much of the action of rotating the hip and waist and aligning the body to take advantage of the virtual draw and to position, power, and direct the punch happen simultaneously instead of in a linear progression, as with the external-style punch, which is another reason why the floating punch can be so fast. Furthermore, unlike the angular external-style punch, which wastes the energy of its backward draw and only gains momentum in the forward throw, the floating punch's circularity has no such break or loss of energy. To the contrary, its (double) circularity guarantees that its momentum constantly gains force, power, and speed throughout its multiple yet almost simultaneous, movements.

A shorter throw and increased force, power, and speed aren't the only advantages of the floating punch over the external-style punch. Another important one is that, unlike the external-style punch, the floating punch does not overtly telegraph itself. If an opponent draws back an arm, you not only can be pretty sure he's going to punch, you can tell what the target and angle of the punch are going to be. But because the floating punch simply launches forward without a highly visible draw and without significant visual clues as to intent, target, and angle, it does not telegraph itself but just launches and impacts with no warning. In addition, the shortness of the floating punch's throw also means that the punch can be effectively thrown at ranges too close for external-style punches to even draw back, much less launch. The external-style jab might seem to be an exception, but again, the jab, while short-range, is a relatively weak punch, while the Tai Chi punch can develop full-body power in equally short—or shorter—distances.

Now let's look at how the muscles of the arm and hand work together to make the fist in the two types of punches. A person using an external-style punch will strongly tighten the muscles of the shoulder and forearm and will partially tighten the muscles of the upper arm. In addition, the external-style fist is tightly clenched. (Figure 6.51) On a simple physical level, the fist is clenched to make it a more dense object with which to strike and, ostensibly, to help protect it from damage. It is not uncommon to see external stylists pound their fists against hard surfaces of one sort or another in order to toughen their fists and to purposefully deform and compress bones—especially the middle knuckle—that might otherwise be broken during a punch into shapes less conducive to breakage.

All this has the effect of making the striking limb denser and outwardly stronger. In essence, the puncher is creating a weight (fist) on the end of a rod (fore-

arm). The weight can be thrust forward for a punch or jab or swung from
various directions, such as from below
for an uppercut or from the side for a
hook. (I'm leaving out the hammer
fist, which would employ the weight
and rod like a hammer striking a nail.
Even though the hammer fist is a strike
with the clenched hand, it isn't techni-

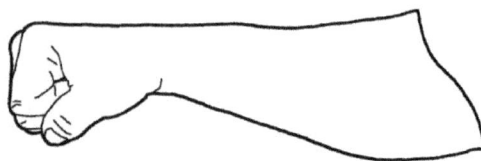

**Figure 6.51** The external-style fist is tightly clenched.

cally a punch because it strikes with the fleshy part at the outside heel of the fist
rather than with the front of the fist, such as knuckles or fingers.)

Something quite different happens in the floating punch. The shoulder and arm
muscles are all relaxed throughout, and the fist itself is loosely held into a hollow fist
shape rather than being clenched. (Figure 6.52) At the instant of impact at the punch's
point of focus, the shoulder muscles remain relaxed, and the forearm muscles tighten
briefly to compact the fist, though in a specialized manner that is not the same as the
clenching and hardening that are characteristic of the external-style punch. We'll discuss that in a moment, but for now, the looseness of the muscles during the punch
allows the arm to retain the flexibility required for Tai Chi's whipping action to snake
through it, both physically and energetically. The brief tightening of the fist at the
moment of impact is tantamount to the tip of a whip hardening instantaneously as
the whipping energy snaking through the whip terminates there, as we looked at previously. And just like the tension at the tip of a whip, the brief tightening of the arm
and fist immediately slacks off upon impact, returning the entire arm to its former
loose state. This not only quickly returns flexibility to the arm, it causes the energy of
the punch to continue straight ahead into the target rather than having some of it rebound into the punching fist, which would both diminish the energy of the punch
and potentially hurt the puncher's fist.

An external stylist might object that a hollow fist that is only slightly tightened cannot
create a dense mass of the fist with which to strike effectively and that a hollow fist would
be more prone to injury. But are these really the case? Let's look at how force and energy
travel down the forearm and through the hand when punching. We'll consider force first
because that is the major motivator of the external-style punch, and its dynamics have
something to say about how force is transmitted by the floating punch.

We've seen how the line of force of a punch travels straight through the forearm
along either the ulna, radius, or both, depending on whether the fist is angled up or

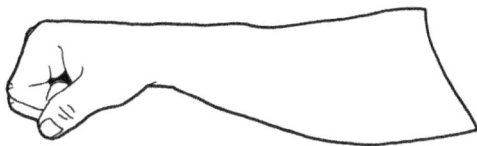

Figure 6.52 The floating fist is relaxed and has a hollow core.

down or not angled. The force then travels through the cluster of bones called the carpals, which are the wrist bones. Then it goes through the metacarpals, or, the bones within the hand, where it terminates at the end of those at the base knuckle joints of the phalanges, or, finger bones. This is a restatement of the line of force noted above that is created by aligning the outside of the forearm, the back of the wrist, and the back of the hand. (Let's ignore, for now, the several other possible fist configurations that do not strictly adhere to this alignment.)

It would be impossible to effectively punch without the force traveling through this exact path, no matter if the punch is external style or floating style. In fact, clenching the fist really only does a couple of things, both unrelated to this line of force. First, it folds the fingers inward, getting them out of the way so that the knuckles can strike. Second, the clenching produces a denser mass with which to strike. But even so, we can see that this mass isn't actually lined up along the axis of force but is offset to one side. (Figure 6.53) What this means is that it is actually possible to punch with the knuckles alone, without forming the fist into a solid mass. While it might seem that the force of a punch is physically augmented to some degree by the denser mass of a clenched fist, the truth is that a clenched fist doesn't weigh any more than a loose fist does—the hand weighs the same whether it is relaxed or clenched.

As shown above, the external-style punch creates this denser mass by clenching the fist into a tight wad of muscle and bone. The floating punch also creates a more solid mass of the fist, but it does it in a completely different way that is directly linked to the arm's relaxed musculature and the fist's hollow center. To understand how it does this, we have to look at how the chi flows through the forearm and hand.

We saw in an earlier section how chi flows into and through open-hand strikes, namely the Lady-like Wrist, the conventional palm strike, and the Roof Tile Palm. Chi likewise flows through the hollow fist, but because of the way the fingers are curled into the palm, the flow doesn't just move down through the inside of the arm, into and through the fingertips, and then back up through the outside of the arm. Instead, the loose curling of the fingers cycles the chi through the fingers and palm, around the fist's hollow core, generating its own small, rotating core of energy. This core is similar to the one that rotates within the chi belly. (Figure 6.54)

As long as the fist is relaxed, this energetic core is really just potential energy, but

as soon as the fist is tightened, the
potential energy becomes much more
energetically dense and powerful. In
*The Wellspring*, I made a distinction
between the ways that external-style
martial arts and the internal-style
martial arts bring chi to bear within
their techniques. That distinction is
important here. Chi is the energy of

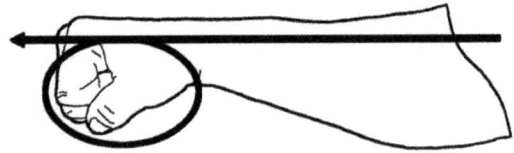

Figure 6.53 Much of the fist does not lie directly along a punch's line of force.

the bioelectromagnetic flow that surrounds nerve channels, and it is created by
stimulating the musculature surrounding those channels. As we've seen, the body
produces whole-body chi in the Conception Vessel via the muscular contractions of
abdominal breathing, which stimulate the enteric plexus to produce a greater bioelectrical charge and attendant bioelectromagnetic flow.

Just as contractions of the muscles surrounding the enteric plexus amplifies the
whole-body chi, contraction of muscles surrounding the meridians in a limb can
amplify chi locally within a limb by stimulating the nerves there to increase their
bioelectric output. This same thing happens when some external force touches your
body and produces electrical signals that travel to your central nervous system as
sensation or pain. It also occurs when you squeeze or clench a muscle, and this is
how the external-style punch generates additional chi in the arm and hand when
punching. Squeezing and hardening the muscles of the forearm and hand creates a
sudden production of chi within those areas, although the chi thus generated is limited to and operates only within the tightened limb. It is like a battery that can produce a sudden, localized, and transient discharge. That discharge might be like a
bolt of lightning that can strike powerfully, but it can strike only in one location
and only briefly. Furthermore, if the discharge is powerful enough, it can deplete
the charge in the battery, and it might take a moment for the chemical reaction to
accumulate additional charge. On the other hand, the steady output of an electric
dynamo can generate and transmit an intense but steady flow of power that does
not require recharging.

So, even though the external-style punch actually does employ chi, though in a
short-lived and strictly localized way within a limb, the very act of tightening the arm
muscles closes off the meridians, momentarily cutting off the greater flow of whole-
body chi through the arm, essentially isolating the striking limb from the body's main
chi circuitry. The floating punch, on the other hand, constantly employs the whole-

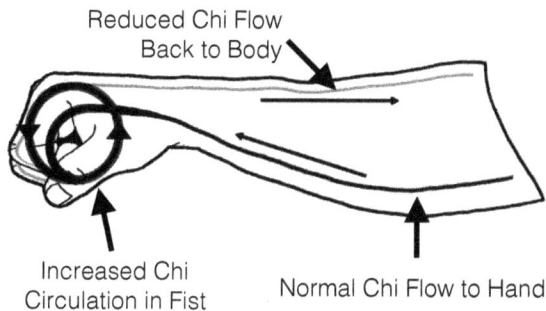

**Figure 6.54** The floating fist showing circulation of energy.

body chi flow, allowing the power of the entire circuitry to be brought to bear in the fist.

Above, we saw how the hollow fist channels that flow into a mini-circuit within the fist. I called this flow a potential energy because it's just cycling there and isn't really doing anything. But the energy can become kinetic by manipulating it—specifically by partially and temporarily blocking the flow to cause a back-up of energy within the fist. This manipulation does not involve wholesale tightening the muscles of the forearm by clenching or hardening them, but by thrusting the presenting knuckle group forward and pulling the tucked fingers inward instead of squeezing them into the palm, in effect, stretching the back of the forearm and the outside surfaces of the carpal and metacarpal areas toward the tips of the phalanges. This stretching action is really a stretching of the fasciae and tendons along the back of the forearm, wrist, and hand, which then automatically pull on the muscles they are attached to, tightening them without tensing or hardening them. It is, if you will, a passive tightening rather than an active squeezing, and it tucks the phalanges into a tighter circle within the palm without clenching the fist and closing off its central hollow core.

Tightening the muscles of the forearm and hand in this way has a significant impact on the chi flowing through the arm. Because the tightening is primarily along the outside of the arm, wrist, hand, and fingers, the muscles of the inner forearm remain relatively relaxed, and the chi continues to flow at full strength into and through them, the inner wrist, and the palm. But this flow quickly loses forward momentum when it cycles through the curled fingers and palm, and it is further blocked from returning completely into the body by the passive tensing of the outer forearm muscles. The more one stretches the fasciae and tendons, the tighter the muscles become, leading to higher degrees of blockage. Any time a meridian is blocked, it causes the chi to back up behind the block, and this holds true with the forearm and hand of the hollow fist, causing the chi flow to build up in the fist and cycle more vigorously and powerfully through it.

The build-up forms a momentary accumulation, not of muscle and bone, but of a small and highly condensed bioelectromagnetic mass. So, instead of producing a localized surge of chi to power a punch that delivers only a physical impact, as does the external-style punch, the floating punch delivers a physical mass accompanied by the powerfully condensed bioelectromagnetic mass cycling in and around the fist. The sharp snap of the floating punch does not have less physical momentum and weight than the physical blow of an external-style punch and so can impart

> The distance that the fist travels in its thrust forward is equal to the sum of all the joints opening. Even though each joint might open up only a fraction of a centimeter, the sum of all these joints opening, extending from the joints in the foot, up the leg, through the hip, up the spine, out the shoulder, through the arm, wrist, and finally propelling the fist forward, is surprisingly large.
>
> —Tina Chunna Zhang[48]

an equivalent physical force, but the Tai Chi punch delivers energy as much as it does physical force. In essence, it violently thrusts a condensed bioelectromagnetic mass, backed by a physical blow, deep into the opponent's biofield and disrupting it. Then, the sudden relaxation and retraction of the fist and arm leave this energy mass embedded inside the opponent's biofield. These are major factors behind the legendary penetrating and explosive power of the floating punch. In fact, this same sort of thing occurs with any expression of fa jin, no matter what body part is used to deliver the force and energy, although the results need not be particularly violent or explosive.

There also is a fundamental difference in how the fist is protected from injury in both the external-style punch and the floating punch. As noted above, the fist of the external-style punch is protected by compacting and hardening it into a mass and by conditioning of, especially, the knuckles. It is not uncommon to see heavy calluses on the knuckles of hard stylists. Such conditioning might make the bones denser, and the calluses might give the knuckles protection, but there is a trade-off in the loss of sensitivity and flexibility in the conditioned hand that could impede whole-body chi flow through it. The hollow Tai Chi fist, however, is protected by its flexibility. Of all the skeletal substructures in the human body, none is more flexible than the hand, and it can withstand a fairly great amount of momentary deformation without serious injury. And looseness is the key to this flexibility. There is an old adage that says that drunk people are more likely to escape serious injury in a car collision than are others because their bodies are more relaxed, and the same might be said of Tai Chi's loose, relaxed fist. You probably won't want to try to verify the former, but you can experiment with the latter by delivering a back fist to a solid wall, first with the back of the fist hardened and then with it relaxed. You'll quickly see that striking with a hardened fist hurts a lot more than striking with a relaxed one, yet the loose fist can deliver a similar impact. And because it doesn't hurt as much, you can hit a little harder.

Before I close this section, I'd like to make a few additional observations about the negative effects of muscular tension and rigidity. Regarding speed, tensed muscles inhibit rapid movement. In a punch, this inhibition is especially crucial at the launch of the punch—the quicker you can launch, the faster and more surprisingly you can get to your target. In addition, in order to change their direction of movement from one trajectory to another, muscle groups have to relax from their movement in the first direction and repurpose themselves for movement in the second direction. We saw this with the dynamics of the external-style punch's draw, but it applies to any number of directional changes. Tai Chi, with its loose musculature, minimizes the time it takes to alter direction, allowing more rapid changes of trajectory.

This rapidity is increased by Tai Chi's circularity. An angular movement has to halt its momentum in one direction before it can move in another, but Tai Chi's circular, twisting movements never actually stop and can almost instantly change direction by simply rotating the angle of the Tai Chi sphere's axis while the sphere remains in motion. But all of this is possible only if the body is loose, flexible, and balanced—in other words: Sung. Further, tension in the shoulders not only inhibits speed and blocks chi flow, it also raises the shoulders and, thus, the body, causing the puncher to break the connection with his root, resulting in loss of power and stability. And finally, tensing the shoulders tends to cause the puncher to form two rigid fists, making the whole area through the shoulders stiff and less mobile, not to mention causing energetic double-weighting within the arms.

Another interesting aspect is that in both the external-style and floating punch, closing the fist vastly reduces or even terminates the energy flowing down the arm by wadding it up there. Manipulating the energy through controlled constrictions in the hands is useful for strikes, but at other times, an open hand is preferable. Using Lady-like Wrists allows the chi flow to be brought unimpeded to a focused and sharp point at the tips of the fingers. Given the electromagnetic nature of chi, the force could potentially extend some greater distance than the hand can actually reach. This finds real-world meaning in many Tai Chi movements. For example,

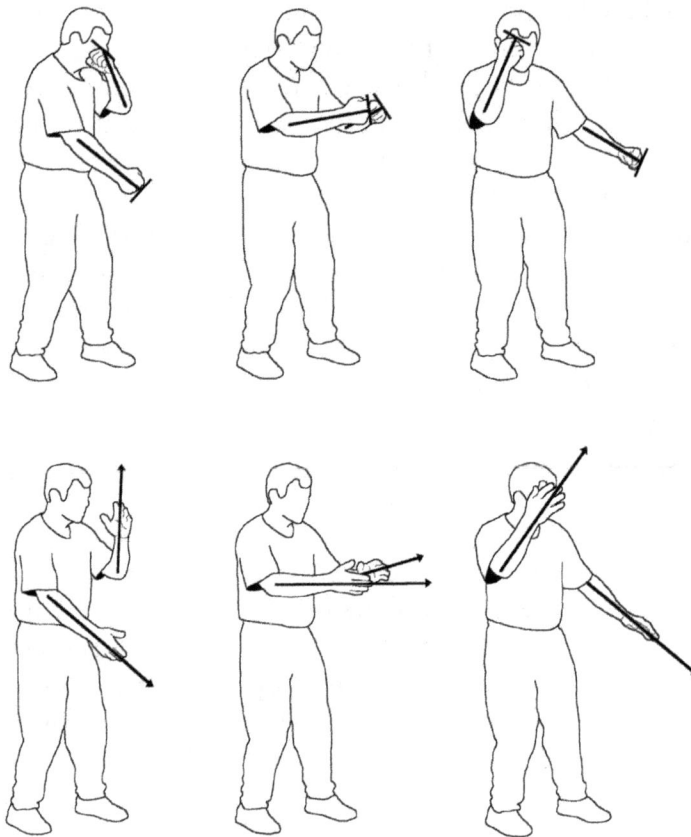

**Figure 6.55** When using Wild Horse Tosses Mane as an arm break, closing the fists (top row) terminates the energy in the fists and forces the movement to use more muscular strength. Open the hands (bottom row) lets the energy extend past the arms, allowing the movement to use greater sense of leverage instead of strength.

when doing Wild Horse Tossing Mane at a slightly more vertical angle than it is normally done in the form, the scissoring arms can be used as an arm break. (Figure 6.55) When scissoring the arms, you can keep the fingers extended or you can close them into fists. If you play with this, you'll notice that keeping the fingers open allows you to feel like you can take advantage of longer leverage during the scissoring than you can if you fold the fingers into fists, and the ability to use a longer lever is an opportunity to bring greater power with less muscular force.

A lot of the dynamics of the punch—both physical and energetic—also apply to open-hand strikes used in other Press movements, such as Brush Knee Twist Step and Maiden Pushing Shuttle, to name just a couple. The main difference is the tool —or particular hand form—one uses with the strike. There are a number of specialized hand forms that have been developed for various martial applications, although Tai Chi tends to employ only a few in its standard styles. These many hand forms are all, in essence, mudras. Mudras are gestures endemic to Buddhism, Taoism, and Hinduism, and although some mudras involve the entire body, most are performed with the hands and fingers. They can be found in many disciplines, such as meditation and the stylized gestures of the classical dances of a number of Eastern cultures, as well as in the martial arts. Mudras often are considered to be symbolic or ritual gestures, but in reality, they are methods to channel chi in specific ways.[49]

There are a great number of mudras in the martial arts, and while most tend to be associated with external styles rather than with Tai Chi, in principle, many can be used with Tai Chi. In the martial arts, mudras are used to facilitate chi flow, as with the Ladylike Wrist, or to condense and channel the chi in specific ways for martial applications, such as basic striking, as with the punch or open-palm strike; deep penetration to seal cavities, as with the Phoenix Eye and Dragon's Head fists; ripping and tearing, as with Eagle Claw and Tiger Claw; or trapping, as with the Crane Wing. But no matter what their specific purpose, they all function similarly to the description I've given above of the chi flow in the fist, and it is simple to extrapolate the flow for each of them. Figure 6.56 depicts a few martial arts mudras to give the reader a sense of their great variety and utility.

As you breathe in, imagine all the energy is going down into the left leg so that you are dis-
tinctly aware of your left leg feeling full, and
different from the rest of the body. Then, while
holding your breath, imagine it flowing around
into the right leg so that when the right leg is full
and complete, the left leg feels hollow and
empty. Then, if you can still hold your breath,
imagine it moving up into your right arm, leaving
the right leg hollow and empty and the right
arm with a full feeling.

—James W. DeMile[50]

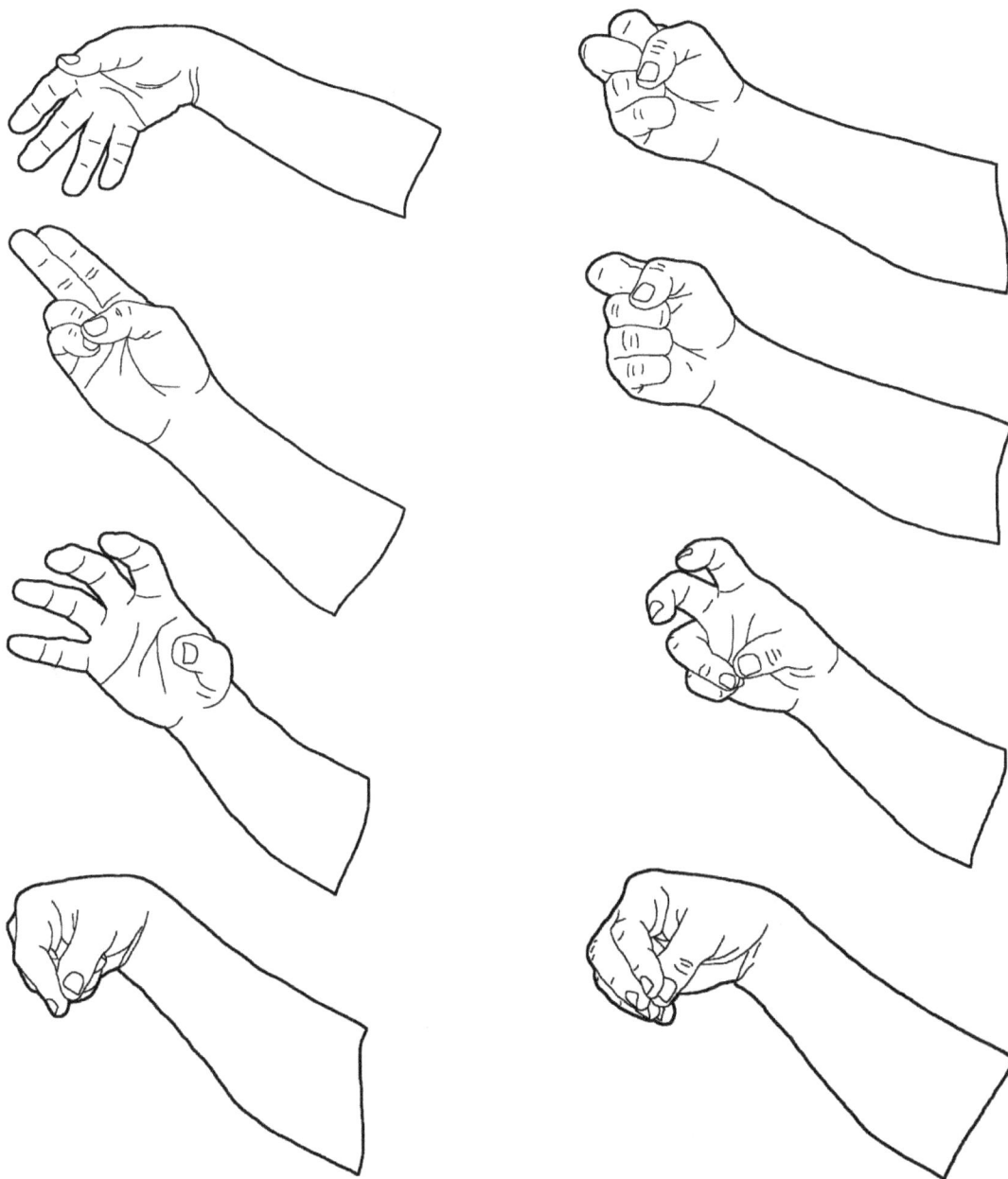

Figure 6.56 A few martial arts mudras: (clockwise from top left) Crane Wing, Dragon's Head, Phoenix Eye Fist, Eagle Claw (Crane Claw), Crane Beak, Eagle's Beak (Praying Mantis Hand), Tiger Claw, Secret Sword.

It is said, that from the Son of Heaven to the common person, cultivating the body is essential to all. Then how does one go about cultivating the body? This is achieved through intrinsic knowledge and abilities. The eyes watch, the ears listen. People speak of acute hearing and clarity of vision. Hands dance and feet tread, one learns martial and intellectual aspects. Upon attaining extraordinary knowledge, one's intention becomes sincere and the mind becomes upright. The mind is master of the body. With upright intention and a sincere mind, feet can step the Five Elements and the hands can dance the Eight Trigrams. If feet and hands act as the Four Symbols applied differently, then intrinsic abilities will return to the origin.

—Wu Kung Cho[51]

# ⑦ Tai Chi, Health, and Beyond

Without self-cultivation, there would be no means of realizing the tao.... Those whose practice is successful both internally and externally reach the highest levels of attainment.

*—Yang Family Forty Chapters*[52]

**The main purpose** of this book has been to explore Tai Chi's physical and energetic dynamics, not its health promoting aspects. That's probably better left to someone with a better grounding in traditional Chinese medicine than I have. But it's hard not to mention health because, in truth, promotion of health is one of the most important reasons to do Tai Chi. Few of us will ever have to fight an opponent, but almost all of us will have to fight the vicissitudes of sickness and aging, so I can't help but make a few comments on the subject of health, particularly since Tai Chi is so well known for endowing its practitioners with vitality and youthfulness of movement, even into older age.

Tai Chi's health promoting aspects are many and varied. The most important is probably that it teaches the practitioner ways to generate and circulate larger amounts of chi than would otherwise occur. As I've said many times earlier, this is due to the specialized process of abdominal breathing, which also is present in other chi-building disciplines, such as meditation and chi kung. This is a better breathing method because it provides deeper and more thorough oxygenation and elimination of carbon dioxide as well as producing a more powerful flow of chi.

The greater density and increased propulsion of the chi have healthful effects. The bioelectrical impulse that gives rise to chi was identified by Dr. Robert O. Becker as being a major factor in the healing of wounds.[53] The amplified chi becomes, in effect, a healing energy that washes through every cell in the body, refreshing and vitalizing them and increasing the body's ability to heal itself and to protect itself from disease. In a sense, it is like continuously bathing the body's cells in a powerful wash of antioxidants.

An antioxidant is a molecule that inhibits the oxidation of other molecules. Oxidation is a chemical reaction that transfers electrons or hydrogen from a substance to an oxidizing agent. Oxidation can produce free radicals: atoms, molecules, or ions that have unpaired valence electrons, which are electrons that occupy an orbit of an atom singly, rather than as a part of an electron pair. The formation of electron pairs is often energetically favorable in creating chemical bonds. Free radicals, on the other hand, can start chemical chain reactions in a cell that cause damage or death to the cell and can even, in worst cases, damage DNA structure, leading to cancer.

Antioxidants terminate these chain reactions by removing free radicals and inhibiting further oxidation. Antioxidants, such as Vitamin C, work on the body at a chemical level by being more readily oxidized than elements of the cell. In a sense, they are like the "sacrificial anodes" placed in large circular metal tanks used to train divers in underwater construction techniques. The walls of such tanks, which are often thirty feet in diameter and fifty or more feet in height, are made of galvanized iron. Construction materials, such as steel beams, are lowered into the tank, where trainee divers then practice welding them into underwater structures like those used in bridge and off-shore oil well construction.

The problem arises because the construction beams are steel, which is harder than the iron of the wall of the tank itself. This turns the entire tank into a gigantic but very low-wattage battery, whose cathode (positive pole) is the steel construction suspended inside and whose anode (negative pole) is the wall of the tank itself. A battery is powered by a migration of electrons from the anode to the cathode—in the case of the tank, from the softer to the harder metal. The effect on the divers is nil, but the process of electrolysis that is created tends to erode the softer metal composing the tank wall, eating it away over time. To prevent this, a block of an even softer metal, such as zinc, is set in the bottom of the tank. This then becomes the battery's anode, and it is this anode that is eaten up instead of the wall of the tank—hence its designation as "sacrificial."

Only further research can demonstrate whether the following idea is valid, but I believe that amplifying the chi, which entails increasing the bioelectrical output of the body's generator and thus increasing the flow of ions throughout the body, might either push free radicals along in the amped-up current or drop additional ions/electrons into the orbits of free radicals, creating electron pairs where there formerly were only unpaired electrons. This would reduce the number of free radicals in the body, thus curtailing their negative effects. Whatever the case might be, it is observably true that people who have practiced chi-enhancing exercises such as Tai Chi exhibit not just greater flexibility and strength than most of their peers as they age, but they also generally retain other positive characteristics, such as a more youthful appearance and greater general health and vitality.

As abdominal breathing amplifies chi and propels it through the Microcosmic and Macrocosmic Orbits, the chi's greater density and power intensify the body's biofield as well as the flow of chi through the body itself. This not only gives the individual a way to neutralize oxidation, thus imparting greater resistance to disease, it also provides a way for the individual to ward off other negative external influences while at the same time allowing deeper sensitivity to positive influences. Great masters are noted for the power of their "presence," and some, such as Wu Ying-hua and her husband, Ma Yueh-liang—for many years the reigning masters of Wu family style—are said to have been able to perceive the biofields, or auras, of other people. For martial purposes, the increased power and awareness of the biofield assists in creating a greater, more substantial wave of energy when the Tai Chi exponent uses, for example, fa jin.

I want to emphasize that this wash of energy cannot be heightened by abdominal breathing alone. It must be accompanied by Sung—the emptying of the muscles and joints of the upper body of tension through proper body alignment and sinking the body's weight and energy into the area below the waist. It doesn't matter how hard you try to pump chi energy—if the body isn't open enough to channel it, it will not flow any more readily. And if your body is tense, you simply cannot feel the flow of chi because the sensing nerves are preoccupied with the sensation of tension.

Thus, Tai Chi also promotes a correct posture that relieves upper body muscles from the strain of using them inappropriately to hold the torso upright. But Sung lends more than just the ability to relieve tension in the upper body. Following the Tai Chi prescription, "Heavy on bottom, light on top," has multiple effects beyond allowing one to loosen the joints and muscles above the waist. The idea here is that although the musculature of the upper body becomes loose, the muscles of the body below the waist become firmer. By this, I don't mean tenser; I mean both stronger and more flexible. This is particularly true of the muscles of the thighs. This leg strength is what the Tai

Chi exponent uses to initiate power in the movements. As one Tai Chi adage has it: The legs are the power of the people, the waist is the commander who directs that power, and the arms and hands are the government and military that express it.

At the same time, the correct body alignments that put the stress of holding up the body onto the legs—the body's foundation—also relieve the knees and ankles, both of which are relatively weak joints despite their importance in supporting the body, from undue stress. Greater strength in the legs leads to improved balance and stability, reducing the chances of falling in older age from being top heavy. But being heavy on bottom and light on top does more in a holistic sense than just promote leg strength and balance. The constant weight shifts and pulsing energetic movements of the leg muscles helps increase vascular circulation and reduce stagnation of the blood in the legs, and the lessened tension in the upper body allows better circulation through the torso, arms, and brain, incidentally relieving stress on the heart.

Loosening the joints and relaxing the muscles of the body also allow the practitioner, over time, to learn to move the body with the fasciae and tendons rather than with the muscles. I don't mean that the Tai Chi expert never uses muscles. Walking around, doing work, or picking up anything requires muscular exertion to some extent, and the alignments of the body and motivation of the fascial trains when using the movements martially can be augmented by muscles used properly. But Tai Chi teaches one to subordinate muscular movement to the stretching and contraction of fasciae and tendons. Most people stiffen as they age, and this isn't so much because their muscles atrophy as because their fasciae and tendons lose their flexibility. But when one learns to use the fasciae and tendons to motivate movement throughout the body, one constantly exercises these structures and keeps them elastic and flexible.

And finally, relaxation of the muscles allows the Tai Chi practitioner to exercise them in a way that is radically different than the squeezing, contraction, and tightening of the muscles normally considered necessary to keep muscles in good shape. Instead, Tai Chi twists the muscles around themselves, around each other, or around their underlying bones. If you think of Tai Chi's corkscrewing, twisting movements, which happen in the limbs as well as in the torso, you'll see what I mean. It is much like the difference between trying to compress a wet dishrag to squeeze out the water as opposed to wringing it out. The latter is much more efficient. And this wringing effect has an important consequence for the muscles. The normal squeezing and contraction of external-style exercise produces a buildup of lactic acid in the muscles, which results in muscle fatigue. But because the twisting of the muscles caused by Tai Chi is accomplished by the stretching and contraction of the fasciae and tendons instead of exerting the muscles themselves, the production of waste products, such as lactic acid, chloride, potassium, and magnesium, to name a few, and the muscle fatigue they cause can be kept to a minimum. In addition, the wringing effect would assist in both circulation of the blood in the muscles and more thoroughly eliminating toxins from them.

One thing that Tai Chi isn't particularly good at is weight loss, per se. But it can assist in regulating the weight by promoting better digestion through the amped-up firing of the neurons in the enteric plexus, which strengthens the peristaltic reflex and keeps food matter moving steadily through the digestive tract.

Many more people practice Tai Chi for its health benefits than for its martial functions, but many of those people simply go through the motions of the Tai Chi movements without activating and mobilizing the chi. For those who are just seeking an energizing, healthful physical exercise, this might be enough because repetitive practice of Tai Chi, even if superficial, will keep one limber and strong. Unfortunately, this sort of practice is a little like going to the movies while wearing a blindfold and ear plugs: One pays the price of admission but reaps few of the more profound benefits. But for those who want more, Tai Chi has a lot to offer.

Over the course of this book, we've spent a great deal of time exploring the dynamics of Tai Chi, first in its physical aspects, then in its energetic ones. This follows the way one acquires Tai Chi. In the beginning, one learns, in a sense, to fashion a container by learning how to perform the Tai Chi form. Tai Chi, done properly, will, through its physical movements, keep the body limber, stronger, and better aligned. But creating the container isn't the end, only the beginning. Once one has created the container, then one can begin to fill it with substance—chi energy. This is where the internal aspect really kicks in. At the basic level, this involves paying attention to the dynamics of the physical movements within one's own body, such as the circularity of the movements and the alignments necessary to make the movements function properly. Over time, as one works on and grows familiar with the movements and integrates them into one's habitual movement patterns in daily life, one begins to learn to relax the musculature of the upper body and, through correct abdominal breathing, amp up the production of chi in the tantien. This, in turn, opens one to awareness of sensations of the chi flow. These sensations, so subtle in the beginning, grow over time, rewarding the attention paid to them. And then one is led to a new avenue of approach, where attention is transformed in intention and one starts to consciously manipulate the chi energy.

Thus one of the core practices of Tai Chi is the strengthening of one's concentration. It takes a special sort of concentration to perform the Tai Chi form. On the surface, when one performs the form, one must think about the form and its many elements, not about extraneous matters such as what you're going to have for dinner or how you're going to solve a problem at work. But one cannot concentrate too deeply on any one aspect of the form—alignments, balance, bodily movements, martial function, chi flow, the energy field, and so forth—or one looses the sense of the others and of the overall flow of the form. Likewise, thinking only of the flow gives short shrift to the separate elements and their purposes and meanings. Instead, the concentration should simultaneously be on the flow of the form and on the form's many elements, and yet it should not be on any of those, either. The concentration should be both pointed and diffuse, and it should shift constantly while remaining focused.

If all of that sounds contradictory—or at least pretty hard to do—maybe it is. Maybe it's as impossible as truly circling the square by just adding more and more facets. The truth, at least for me, is that I can't hold all the elements and the flow in my consciousness at one time but must focus here and there throughout my practice. I'm not sure that anyone can concentrate on all the elements, anyway, since certain movements can be used for radically opposing functions in which force and energy operate quite differently, and by the time you've thought of or performed one aspect, the movement is finished, and you move on to the next one. Instead, I try to think of this or that about the form and its movements and try to ignore the extraneous thoughts that constantly run through my head. In the end, I can only hope that, over time and through multiple repetitions of the form, I touch on as many of the elements in their disparate aspects as I can while I attempt to integrate them into the flow.

The true benefits of Tai Chi lie in the strengthening and conscious regulation of chi, which, as I've said before, is intimately tied to its functioning as a martial art. This isn't because learning to defend oneself is healthful, per se, but because the functional aspects of the movements provide practical guidance that specifically teaches the practitioner how to move chi energy around within the body in different ways. Of course, it is possible to apply the Tai Chi movements in a strictly physical—external—manner. Tai Chi is, after all, a type of kung fu, and many of its movements and applications can be found in external styles. But the Tai Chi exponent can gain tremendous power by synchronizing the physical movements with the flow of chi through the meridians and with the many possible permutations of the circular/oval rotations of the body's energy fields. Together, the physical and energy dynamics produce exponentially greater results than either could alone, and they also increase and direct the conjoined force and energy in ways that allow the energy to exceed the bounds of the container that once held it, opening one to the universal energies that surround us.

> The elixir of long life is within the body
> That we may restore our primal purity.
> Spiritual cultivation brings great virtue.
> Regulate it well and the ch'i and body will be whole.
> For ten thousand years, chant the praises of eternal spring;
> Truly the mind is the genuine article.
>
> —Chang San-feng[54]

Tai Chi and other chi-building exercises are forms of true alchemy, where the practitioner attempts to refine and condense his or her spiritual being in the retort of the body via the energy (heat/chi) generated by abdominal breathing. The goal is to create the Elixir of Life or Pill of Immortality, often falsely believed by many would-be and materialistically minded alchemists who mistook this spiritual practice as a chemical operation performed with laboratory equipment and to be an external substance that one consumes to attain spiritual or physical immortality. Even more-materialistically minded alchemists thought, even more erroneously, that it is a process to produce gold from base metals. True alchemy is a physiological and psychological process that attempts to refine the lead of the cruder, base elements or aspects of one's being into something more pure: the gold of enlightenment. It can produce spiritual results by helping cleanse the system of impurities and impediments—be they physical, emotional, or spiritual—eventually allowing the strengthened bioenergies and purified spirit to rise up the Governing Vessel, emerge from the Crown Chakra, and merge with the greater spiritual presences of the universe. This idea is at the foundations of a number of religions. In the Buddhist tradition, for example, this state is called Nirvana; in Taoism, it is merging with the Tao.

For me, the most important benefit of Tai Chi is its use as a tool for self-development. It is an alchemy that helps me open to my inner workings and make me more sensitive to my surroundings in ways I had no idea existed before I took it up. Tai Chi is a fascinating discipline: fascinating to perform, fascinating to apply, and fascinating to ponder. And my fascination with it has only grown the longer I've practiced.

We've come a long way in this book, but any theory of Tai Chi is bound to be faulty and incomplete, not just because the art's concepts are so manifold and difficult to describe, but because every time you look at anything about Tai Chi, you see something hiding deeper in the background. And the deeper you look, the more Tai Chi continues to open new vistas of interlinking functions and operations all regulated through a brilliant set of principles that can greatly enhance life on many levels—levels that, in turn, go deeper still.

Much of that depth may be beyond my reach or ken, but even so, I hope I've managed through this book's many words and illustrations to convey some useful information along with my personal fascination with the subject. These are the thoughts I have and tenets I hold about Tai Chi—at least at this moment. But I'm still learning, and all this could change or be further refined in a moment thanks to new evidence. For now, though, thanks for listening.

# Appendix

# Footnotes

1 Hexagram 2, Moving Line 2, *The I Ching or Book of Changes*, Richard Wilhelm (trans., rendered into English by Cary F. Baynes) (Bollingen Series XIX, Princeton University Press, 1950), p. 13.

2 Campbell, Joseph, *The Hero with a Thousand Faces* (Bollingen Series XVII, Princeton University Press, 1949), p. 42.

3 *Wikipedia* entry, "Tai chi," http://en.wikipedia.org/wiki/T%27ai_chi_ch%27uan.

4 Jou, Tsung Hwa, *The Tao of Tai-Chi Chuan* (Charles E. Tuttle Co., 1980), p. 226-227.

5 "Yang Family Manuscripts Copied by Shen Chia-chen," in *Tai Chi Touchstones: Yang Family Secret Transmissions*, Douglas Wile (comp. & trans.) (Sweet Chi Press, 1983), p. 84.

6 "The Secret of the Eighteen Loci," from "Nine Secret Transmissions on T'ai-chi Ch'üan," by Wu Meng-hsia, in *Tai Chi Touchstones: Yang Family Secret Transmissions*, Douglas Wile (comp. and trans.) (Sweet Chi Press, 1983), p. 79.

7 Cirlot, J. E., *A Dictionary of Symbols* (Jack Sage, trans.) (Philosophical Library, 1962), p. 15.

8 Wu, Kung Cho, *Wu Style Tai Chi Chuan* (Doug Woolidge, trans.) (International Wu Style Tai Chi Federation, 2006), p. 38.

9 Huang, Wen-shan, *Fundamentals of T'ai Chi Ch'uan* (South Sky Book Company, 1982), p. 53.

10 Cheng, Man-ching, from a translation of "Master Cheng's Thirteen Chapters on T'ai-chi ch'uan," (1975) in *Ta'i-chi Touchstones: Yang Family Secret Transmissions*, Douglas Wile (comp. and trans.) (Sweet Chi Press, 1983), p. 18.

11 *Wikipedia* entry, "Torque," http://en.wikipedia.org/wiki/Torque.

12 Wang, Tsung-yüeh, "Wang Tsung-yüeh's Treatise on T'ai-chi ch'üan," in *T'ai-chi Touchstones: Yang Family Secret Transmissions*, Douglas Wile (comp. and trans.) (Sweet Chi Press, 1983), p. 134.

13 Wu, Meng-hsia, "The Secret of the Free Circle," from "Nine Secret Transmissions on T'ai-chi ch'üan," in *T'ai-chi Touchstones: Yang Family Secret Transmissions*, Douglas Wile (comp. and trans.) (Sweet Chi Press, 1983), p. 77.

14 Yang, Lu-ch'an, "Yang Lu-ch'an's Commentary to the T'ai-chi ch'üan Classic," in *T'ai-chi Touchstones: Yang Family Secret Transmissions*, Douglas Wile (comp. and trans.) (Sweet Chi Press, 1983), p. 109.

15 Jou, Tsung Hwa, *The Tao of Tai-Chi Chuan* (Charles E. Tuttle, Co., 1980), p. 80-81.

16 *Wikipedia* entry, "Tai chi," http://en.wikipedia.org/wiki/T%27ai_chi_ch%27uan.

17 Wang, Tsung-yüeh, "Wang Tsung-yüeh's Treatise on T'ai-chi ch'üan," in *T'ai-chi Touchstones: Yang Family Secret Transmissions*, Douglas Wile (comp. and trans.) (Sweet Chi Press, 1983), p. 119.

18 Jou Tsung Hwa, *The Tao of Tai-Chi Chuan* (Charles E. Tuttle Co., 1980) p. 143.

19 *Wikipedia* entry, "Golden ratio," http://en.wikipedia.org/wiki/Golden_ratio.

20 Zeising, Adolf, *Neue Lehre van den Proportionen des meschlischen Körpers* (1854), preface, from *Wikipedia* entry, "Golden ratio," http://en.wikipedia.org/wiki/Golden_ratio.

21 *Wikipedia* entry, (Taijitu," http://en.wikipedia.org/wiki/Taijitu.

22 Li, I-yü, "Song of the Circulation of Ch'i," from "The Writings of Li I-yü," in *Lost T'ai-chi Classics from the Late Ch'ing Dynasty*, by Douglas Wile (State University of New York Press, 1996), p. 55.

23 Zi, Nancy, *The Art of Breathing: Thirty Simple Exercises for Improving Your Performance and Well-being* (Bantam Books, 1986), p. 4.

24 Cirlot, J. E., *A Dictionary of Symbols* (Jack Sage, trans.) (Philosophical Library, 1962), p. 31.

25 Yang, Ch'eng-fu, "An Explanation of Wang Tsung-yüeh's Original Introduction," from "Yang Ch'eng-fu's Self-Defense Applications of T'ai-chi ch'üan," in *T'ai-chi Touchstones: Yang Family Secret Transmissions*, Douglas Wile (comp. and trans.) (Sweet Chi Press, 1983), p. 109.

26 *Wikipedia* entry, "Tendon," http://en.wikipedia.org/wiki/Tendon.

27 After Thomas Myers, *Anatomy Trains: Myofascial Meridians for Manual and Movement Therapists* (Churchill Livingstone, 2014).

28 I refer the reader to Trevor Aung Than's article, "TCM meridians and fascia: what does it have to do with the internal arts?" http://circusconditioning. com/?p=275.

29 Wu, Yu-hsiang, "Expositions of Insights into the Practice of the Thirteen Postures," in *The Essence of T'ai Chi Ch'uan: The Literary Tradition*, Benjamin Pang Jeng Lo, Martin Inn, Robert Amacker, Susan Foe (trans. and eds.) (North Atlantic Books, 1985), p. 53.

30 Becker, Robert O., M.D., and Gary Selden, *The Body Electric: Electromagnetism and the Foundation of Life* (Quill, 1985), p. 92.

31 *Wikipedia* entry, "Hydraulic analogy," http://en.wikipedia.org/wiki/Hydraulic_analogy.

32 *Wikipedia* entry, "Fundamental interactions," http://en.wikipedia.org/wiki/Fundamental_interaction.

33 Yang, Jwing-Ming, *Taijiquan Theory: The Root of Taijiquan* (YMAA Publications Center, 2003), p. 93.

34 Gershon, Michael D., M.D., *The Second Brain: A Groundbreaking New Understanding of Nervous Disorders of the Stomach and Intestines* (Quill, 1998), p. 17-18.

35 Becker, Robert O., M.D., and Gary Selden, *The Body Electric: Electromagnetism and the Foundation of Life* (Quill, 1985), see index for entries on "Current of Injury" and "Electricity."

36 The reference work I consult most on the meridian system is *Acupuncture Medicine: Its Historical and Clinical Background*, by Yoshiaki Omura, Sc.D., M.D. (Japan Publications, 1982), but there are many excellent works on this topic of study.

37 *Wikipedia* entry, "Van de Graaff generator," http://en.wikipedia.org/wiki/Van_de_Graaff_generator, and *Wiki Commons*, http://en.wikipedia.org/ wiki/Van_de_Graaff_generator#/media/File:Van_de_Graaff_Generator.svg.

38 *Wikipedia* entry, "Van de Graaff generator," http://en.wikipedia.org/wiki/Van_de_Graaff_generator.

39 Becker, Robert O., M.D., and Gary Selden, *The Body Electric: Electromagnetism and the Foundation of Life* (Quill, 1985), p. 98.

40 Becker, Robert O., M.D., and Gary Selden, *The Body Electric: Electromagnetism and the Foundation of Life* (Quill, 1985), p. 234-235.

41 *Wikipedia* entry, "Brain," http://en.wikipedia.org/wiki/Brain.

42 Yang, Jwing-Ming, *Advanced Yang Style Tai Chi Chuan: Volume One, Tai Chi Theory and Tai Chi Jing* (Yang's Martial Arts Academy, 1986), p. 28.

43 Becker, Robert O., M.D., and Gary Selden, *The Body Electric: Electromagnetism and the Foundation of Life* (Quill, 1985), p. 243.

44 *Wikipedia* entry, "Wave," http://en.wikipedia.org/wiki/Wave.

45 Cirlot, J. E., *A Dictionary of Symbols* (Jack Sage, trans.) (Philosophical Library, 1962), p. 293-294.

46 *Wikipedia* entry, "Torus," http://en.wikipedia.org/wiki/Torus.

47 Yang, Jwing-Ming, *Advanced Yang Style Tai Chi Chuan: Volume One, Tai Chi Theory and Tai Chi Jing* (Yang's Martial Arts Academy, 1986), p. 74.

48 Zhang, Tina Chunna, Frank Allen, *Classical Northern Wu Style Tai Ji Quan: The Fighting Art of the Manchurian Palace Guard* (Blue Snake Books, 2006), p. 31.

49 *Wikipedia* entry, "Mudra," http://en.wikipedia.org/wiki/Mudra.

50 DeMile, James W., *Floating Punch* (3rd edition) (Tao of Wing Chun Do Publications, 1979), p. 10.

51 Wu, Kung Cho, *Wu Style Tai Chi Chuan* (Doug Woolidge, trans.) (International Wu Style Tai Chi Chuan Federation, 2006), p. 40.

52 "An Explanation of the Three Levels of the Spiritual and Martial in T'ai-chi," from "Yang Family Forty Chapters," in *Lost T'ai-chi Classics from the Late Ch'ing Dynasty*, Douglas Wile (State University of New York Press, 1996) p. 75.

53 Becker, Robert O., M.D., and Gary Selden, *The Body Electric: Electromagnetism and the Foundation of Life* (Quill, 1985), see index for entries on "Current of Injury" and "Electricity."

54 "The Legacy of Chang San-feng," from "Yang Family Forty Chapters," in *Lost T'ai-chi Classics from the Late Ch'ing Dynasty*, Douglas Wile (State University of New York Press, 1996), p. 86.

# Bibliography

Becker, Robert O., M.D., and Gary Selden, *The Body Electric: Electromagnetism and the Foundation of Life* (Quill, 1985).

Campbell, Joseph. *The Hero with a Thousand Faces* (Bollingen Series XVII, Princeton University Press, 1949).

Cheng, Man Ch'ing. *Cheng Tzu's Thirteen Treatises on T'ai Chi Ch'uan* (Benjamin Pang Jeng Lo, Martin Inn, trans.) (North Atlantic Books, 1985).

Cirlot, J. E. *A Dictionary of Symbols* (Jack Sage, trans.) (Philosophical Library, 1962).

DeMile, James W. *Floating Punch* (3rd edition) (Tao of Wing Chun Do Publications, 1979).

Docherty, Dan. *Tai Chi Chuan: Decoding the Classics for the Modern Martial Artist* (The Crowood Press, 2009).

Dow, Christopher. *The Wellspring: An Inquiry into the Nature of Chi* (Phosphene Publishing Co., 2008).

Gershon, Michael D., M.D. *The Second Brain: A Groundbreaking New Understanding of Nervous Disorders of the Stomach and Intestines* (Quill, 1998).

Huang, Wen-Shan. *Fundamentals of Tai Chi Ch'uan* (South Sky Book Co., 1982).

*The I Ching or Book of Changes*, Richard Wilhelm (trans., rendered into English by Cary F. Baynes) (Bollingen Series XIX, Princeton University Press, 1950).

Jou, Tsung Hwa. *The Tao of Tai-Chi Chuan* (Charles E. Tuttle Co., 1980).

Lo, Benjamin Pang Jeng, Martin Inn, Robert Amacker, Susan Foe. *The Essence of T'ai Chi Chuan: The Literary Tradition* (North Atlantic Books, 1985).

Myers, Thomas. *Anatomy Trains: Myofascial Meridians for Manual and Movement Therapists* (Churchill Livingstone, 2014).

Omura, Yoshiaki, Sc.D., M.D. *Acupuncture Medicine: Its Historical and Clinical Background* (Japan Publications, 1982).

Wile, Douglas. *Lost T'ai-chi Classics from the Late Ch'ing Dynasty* (State University of New York Press, 1996).

Wile, Douglas (comp. & ed). *T'ai-chi Touchstones: Yang Family Secret Transmissions* (Sweet Chi Press, 1983).

Wu, Kung Cho. *Wu Style Tai Chi Chuan* (Doug Woolidge, trans.) (International Wu Style Tai Chi Chuan Federation, 2006).

Wu, Ying-hua, Ma Yeuh-liang. *Wu Style Taichichuan: Forms, Concepts and Application of the Original Style* (Shanghai Book Co., Ltd., 1988).

Yang, Jwing-Ming. *Advanced Yang Style Tai Chi Chuan: Volume I, Tai Chi Theory and Tai Chi Jing* (Yang's Martial Arts Academy, 1986).

Yang, Jwing-Ming. *Tai Chi Secrets of the Wu Style* (Ymaa Publication Center, 2002).

Yang, Jwing-Ming. *Taijiquan Theory* (YMAA Publication Center, 2003).

Zhang, Tina Chunna, Frank Allen. *Classical Northern Wu Style Tai Ji Quan: The Fighting Art of the Manchurian Palace Guard* (Blue Snake Books, 2006).

Zi, Nancy. *The Art of Breathing: Thirty Simple Exercises for Improving Your Performance and Well-being* (Bantam Books, 1986).

Phosphene Publishing Company
publishes books and DVDs relating to literature,
history, the paranormal, film, spirituality, and the
martial arts.

For other great titles, visit
phosphenepublishing.com

www.ingramcontent.com/pod-product-compliance
Lightning Source LLC
Chambersburg PA
CBHW080458110426
42742CB00017B/2929